The Development and Exploitation of Empirical Birthweight Standards

To Glennis, Sylvaine,
Aileen, Antonia and Eva,
and Jon-Paul

The Development and Exploitation of Empirical Birthweight Standards

Roy Carr-Hill

Centre for Health Economics
Institute for Research in the Social Sciences
University of York

and

Colin Pritchard

MRC Medical Sociology Unit
Institute of Medical Sociology
Westburn Road
Aberdeen

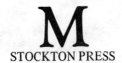

STOCKTON PRESS

First published 1985

Published by
THE MACMILLAN PRESS LTD
Houndmills, Basingstoke, Hampshire RG21 2XS
and London
Companies and representatives
throughout the world

Printed in Great Britain, at the University Press, Oxford

British Library Cataloguing in Publication Data
Carr-Hill, Roy
The development and exploitation of
empirical birthweight standards.
1. Birth weight
I. Title   II. Pritchard, Colin
618.92'01   RJ252
ISBN 0-333-37297-2

Published in the USA and Canada by STOCKTON PRESS, 1985
15 East 26th Street, New York, N.Y. 10010

ISBN 0-943818-07-9

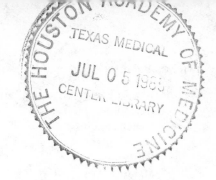

Contents

SECTION 3 THE DERIVATION OF BIRTHWEIGHT STANDARDS

x   *Contents*

Foreword

by
Ian MacGillivray,
Regius Professor,
Department of Obstetrics and Gynaecology
University of Aberdeen

There has been interest in the birthweight of babies in Aberdeen ever since the pioneering work of that outstanding obstetrician and father of epidemiological and social obstetrics, Sir Dugald Baird. The focus of research has tended to be on the extremes of birthweight. Whilst both low and high birthweight can lead to problems for the baby, it is especially low birthweight babies often born into under-privileged situations who account for elevated perinatal mortality and morbidity. Although this is particularly the case in developing countries, it remains an issue in developed countries. Whatever the location, however, the crucial problem is the appropriate procedure which should be used in the assessment of birthweight.

The need for standardised birthweight scores which make the recognition of deviations from the normal possible, has long been appreciated. It was, once again, under the inspiration and guidance of Sir Dugald Baird that A.M. Thomson and W.Z. Billewicz, two non-obstetricians, developed the well-known and widely used Aberdeen standards of birthweight. These standards were based on the population of births, excluding some stillbirths and multiple births, for the city of Aberdeen, which is at sea-level. Another well-known standard of birthweight was developed by Lubchenco in Denver, Colorado, which is about a mile above sea-level. Again, Lubchenco's standards are widely used throughout the world and both these standards serve a useful purpose. It was, however, obvious that neither of these standards should really be applied to any population other than the ones from which they were derived. Indeed, their application to other populations could be erroneous and misleading: for example, the application of the Aberdeen standards to the Asian population in Birmingham has been queried.

The problem of applicability has occasionally prompted the search for standards which would be more universally appropriate. The present authors (once again two non-obstetricians) took up this challenge, encouraged by their colleagues in the Sociological, Obstetrical and Gynaecological Research Group in Aberdeen. They pursued this objective through the several layers of theory formulations, model specifications and difficulties of measurement. They concluded that it was impossible to produce one set of standards which would be applicable world-wide. This conclusion led them to address themselves to the problem of identifying the factors which should be taken into account in devising standards for any population and thereby they establish a model on which appropriate local standards could be developed. This theoretical model and the approach they recommend to analysing the data will make it possible for anyone who has the requisite population data to derive their own standards.

It must, however, be emphasised that this is a theoretical model and that the standards developed in chapters 7, 8 and 9 are for illustrative purposes and relate only to the population on which they are based. Thus, in demonstrating this model, the authors have drawn on the total hospital population coming into the Maternity Hospital in Aberdeen, not only from the city but also from the surrounding country, in order to maximise numbers for analysis. A set of standards specifically for the Aberdeen City and District population is being produced separately.

This book represents a major and important piece of work which should have wide application and will have great clinical importance when the method is applied to particular local populations. Ethnic and other local differences in factors which affect birthweight will then be taken into account. It will become possible to assess the impact of various adverse factors on the specific birthweight distributions and thus to direct resources more effectively to their correction. The authors have performed a great service to the obstetric world in producing this model which others can apply to their own populations. Standards developed locally in this way will facilitate their more confident use and thus enhance their clinical value.

The development of the analysis may appear complicated to some obstetricians. Nevertheless, the authors' basic argument is obviously of crucial importance to them in that it highlights the necessity of developing standards for their own populations and provides a definitive account of how the task should be undertaken. It is for this reason that this book should be read world-wide by obstetricians and paediatricians as well as by statisticians and administrators, so that the local standards can be developed and applied to birthweight distributions with all that this implies for clinical care.

Preface and Acknowledgements

For all concerned, the weight of a baby at birth is pregnant with meaning. Every mother remembers the birthweight of her baby; for the obstetrician, the weight provides a final commentary on the course of the pregnancy; and for the neonatal paediatrician it is one of the many factors (s)he takes into account in deciding which babies are in need of special care immediately after birth.

For both lay and professional understanding of birthweight, it is the *relative* birthweight that is important. The mother is interested in whether this baby is heavier or lighter than her previous baby or that of her neighbour or sister. The medical professional, assessing the health of the baby or the course of the pregnancy, interprets the birthweight in terms of some notion of what the *normal* baby *ought* to weigh, and it is her or his *interpretation* that informs the corresponding medical practice.

Because of the importance of the medical assessment of birthweight, there has been a long history of scientific attempts to provide an objective basis for the judgement of what the normal baby ought to weigh. This has usually involved establishing a set of 'standards' for birthweight. This monograph is intended as a contribution to that tradition, concentrating on the methodological issues involved in the derivation and use of *any* set of standards.

Whilst, however, this monograph is primarily intended to be of use to the medical community, much of the argument will interest epidemiologists and statisticians more generally. First, the problem of defining an appropriate population is one of their central concerns; second, the necessity of a formal model and the difficulty of developing an identifiable model is a constant headache for them; and third, success of a particular strategy for coping with complex interactions and multi-collinearities is always of interest. Similarly, as birthweight standards are used clinically for the *management* of the neonate, the argument should also be of interest to local health administrators.

Our motivation in undertaking a detailed examination of the derivation and potential use of birthweight standards was an unease at the increasing reliance upon estimates of normal birthweight based upon statistical manipulation in the absence of a substantive model of fetal growth. Nevertheless, we are certain that statistical methods do have a considerable contribution to make in this area; and indeed, we would argue that the derivation and appropriateness of such standards has to be considered within a statistical framework. For us, whilst the *use* of standards of normal birthweight does not necessarily require statistical acumen, the very concept of 'normal' birthweight depends on the statistical properties of the underlying distributions of birthweight and factors known to be associated with birthweight (commonly length of gestation, infant sex and maternal parity). Moreover, the assessment of normality in the light of variations in the factors must depend upon their inter-relationships within the framework of a coherent formal model.

It is, of course, well known that birthweight cannot be assessed independently of the gestation at which the baby was born and that boys are 'naturally' heavier than girls. There has also been a wide variety of studies showing the difference between first- and later-born babies, the importance of the mother's own height and weight, and the effect of a whole host of other factors on the likely birth-weight (see chapter 3). What prompted us to investigate this set of inter-relation-ships further was the lack of a coherent model with which to establish a hier-archy between this wide range of determining factors (chapter 4). Our initial analyses of the extensive data available in the Aberdeen Maternity and Neonatal Data Bank (Carr-Hill and Pritchard, 1983) only reinforced our belief that the apparent simplicity of deriving birthweight scores 'standardised' for the deter-mining factors masked complexities in both the research use and clinical inter-pretation of the standards (chapter 2). We explore these theoretical complexities in some detail in our attempt to develop a model in chapter 5.

We therefore went on to investigate the inter-relationships between the different sets of factors in order to see whether a universal model could be developed in the second section. The empirical analysis here is based on the data from the Aberdeen Maternity and Neonatal Data Bank (chapter 6) and the detailed results of our analysis are reported in chapters 7 and 8. It is our finding that 'circumstances change cases' that has prompted us to develop the original article length analyses into a full-length monograph in order to present a con-vincing argument for the necessity of developing locally based birthweight standards appropriate for particular populations. We show how standards deve-loped in this way are useful in both the clinical and research context in the final section of the book (chapters 9, 10 and 11).

We have been very lucky in the continual support given to the whole enter-prise by our own households, especially during the period when one of the authors was peripatetic between Aberdeen and York.

We have been supported throughout our work by the MRC Medical Sociology Unit in Aberdeen to which Colin Pritchard is still attached. Roy Carr-Hill would also like to thank the Centre for Health Economics at York who allowed him time off to finish the book.

We owe a considerable intellectual debt to Professor Ian MacGillivray, Drs Doris Campbell and Marion Hall of the Aberdeen Maternity Hospital who set us off on the trail of a universal set of birthweight standards and have since provided continual advice, encouragement and help, especially in our search for understanding. The monograph has benefited considerably from the comments not only of our Aberdeen colleagues mentioned above but also of several individuals upon whom we inflicted the original manuscript. We received very helpful comments from Professor Dobbing of Manchester University, Steve Duffey of the Clinical Research Centre and the un-named referee to whom Macmillan sent the original manuscript.

The empirical analysis has been based around a set of data chosen according to particular criteria and modified in various ways. The extraction of the basic data from the Aberdeen Maternity Hospital and Neonatal Data Bank was accomplished for us by Mike Samphier and some of the last-minute modifications that were required were performed by Guy Muhleman. Sheena Johnson and Pat Will helped considerably with checking the tables and proofreading.

We have been particularly fortunate in the kindness shown to us by the secretaries who have been involved in this work. Muriel Burnett, Lorraine Gibb and Glennis Whyte all helped at various stages; but our main debt here is to Jeanette Thorne who orchestrated the typing of both the original and revised manuscripts. We would also like to mention the superb artwork done by the Medical Illustrations Section of Aberdeen Maternity Hospital.

Finally we would like to record our debt to Barbara Thomson. Quite simply, without her, we would not have done it.

In view of the long list above, we must conclude by stressing that all errors are our own.

York and Aberdeen, 1984   R.A.C.-H.
                                                                          C.W.P.

SECTION 1

Introduction and birthweight trends since 1950

1
Introduction

THE MAIN ARGUMENT

This monograph is focussed around the assessment of birthweight for gestation whether for clinical or research purposes and, in particular, on the development and utility of birthweight standards. There have, of course, been many studies of the distribution of birthweight among different population groups and of a wide range of factors affecting variations in birthweight. This monograph concentrates on more methodological issues. Thus a recurrent theme is the argument for the development and utility of specific and targetted population based empirical standards, and we propose and pursue a particular analytic strategy which could be used on any reasonably large data set once the population base has been chosen. The whole argument of the monograph is illustrated using appropriate statistical techniques, with material from the Aberdeen Maternity and Neo Natal Data Bank (Samphier and Thompson, 1982).

The argument developed out of the detailed comparison of birthweight surveys which reveals only broad similarities in mean birthweight for gestation and the relative magnitude and significance of effects. Two recent Scottish examples are Forbes and Smalls (1983) based on Glasgow births and Carr-Hill and Pritchard (1983) based on the Aberdeen data used in this monograph. Both papers conclude by arguing the need for standards appropriate to particular populations at particular times.

We take the position that the problems discussed by those authors arise from the absence of a universally acceptable model of fetal growth. This monograph takes that argument further to show that, in the present state of ignorance, the fetal growth process cannot be isolated or identified both because of the unknown degree of interdependence between fetal weight and the gestational age at onset of labour and because of the empirical difficulty of arriving at a precise estimate of gestation independent of the characteristics of the neonate.

It is argued that there is thus a systematic ambiguity between the fetal growth process and observed distributions of birthweight for gestational age. This ambiguity also implies that any given population is potentially composed of an unknown mix of two or more different groups who are different in respect of

3

their typical fetal growth process. This same ambiguity is the reason why the central section of this monograph is devoted to a detailed discussion of how birthweight standards appropriate to a particular population can be derived empirically, illustrated by reference to the Aberdeen population.

Accepting an empirical, essentially descriptive approach means that analysis must proceed carefully, taking account of the story told by the data at each step. As will be apparent in the ensuing chapters, this monograph takes the implications of being an empiricist very seriously. This does not, of course, mean that there is no model at all. Indeed, without some structure to guide inference, it would be impossible to exploit the data, other than to provide a statistical account of the variance of birthweight in a particular population.

The appropriateness of even a loose structure depends on the use to which the standards will be put. For this reason, some prior consideration of the nature of birthweight standards is needed and should be taken into account at all stages of the argument.

CLINICAL AND RESEARCH USE OF STANDARDS

The need to diagnose light- or heavy-for-dates babies and the usefulness of knowing about the normal range of birthweight in a particular population is one of the motives behind the numerous birthweight surveys in the literature. But the *clinical* and *research* uses of standards differ and have different implications for the form of appropriate standards. Some of the salient differences are summarised in table 1.1.

Table 1.1 Clinical and research standards

	Clinical	*Research*
Focus of concern	(a) 'Individual'	Groups defined by research interest
Factors used in defining standards	(b) A few readily measured factors	According to research interests. . .
Form of standards	(c) In readily available form	May be complexly calculated
Treatment of deviations from standards	(d) Statistical significance of deviations not so important as 'practical' significance	Statistical tests generally used in the evaluation of research hypotheses
The concept of 'normal'	(e) Defines the population used for deriving standards	Defined by the population being researched

Focus of concern

The clinical use of birthweight standards tends to be for the assessment of the growth of individual babies; the question being asked is whether a particular baby's growth has departed from the normal up to the time of its birth. This is then used as one of the bases for the prognosis and in determining the appropriate treatment of the new born infant. In research use, standards provide a convenient way of controlling for factors whose effects are not of immediate concern in the research but whose effects may mask the importance of other factors which are of interest (see chapter 5). Research use tends to focus interest on subgroups of the population sharing the attributes whose effects are being researched as, for example, in chapters 10 and 11.

Factors defining standards

For clinical use the factors defining standards are bound to be constrained by the information which is likely to be easily accessible to the clinician at the time an assessment of the fetal growth of a particular baby is to be made. In practice, this means a restriction to the kinds of data which can be routinely collected. Furthermore, as commented immediately below, the more factors incorporated in standards the more complex the assessment of individual babies becomes. A researcher, on the other hand, may wish to take account of rather more factors. However, retrospective research will also be constrained to the information which is routinely collected. Even prospective research is constrained by the practicalities of collecting such data. The variety of factors that have been considered in other studies are illustrated in chapters 3 and 4.

Form of standards

In a clinical setting, the use of readily understood 'look-up' tables (e.g. those derived by Thomson *et al.*, 1968) or the nomograms produced by Altman and Coles (1980) are especially appropriate. They enable swift and accurate assessments based on relatively few important factors to be made. The researcher, with the aid of computers, can perform complex statistical operations using many factors, so the standards do not need to be in a readily accessible form. The emphasis in this monograph on the development and exploitation of research standards accounts for the form in which the standards are presented in chapters 7 and 8.

Deviation from the standard

The evaluation of the significance of departures from the 'normal' represented by the 'standard' are also likely to differ for clinicians and researchers. For example, in the Aberdeen survey discussed later, the mean weight of first-born boys at 32 weeks gestation is 1843 g with a standard deviation of 321.8 g. If a statistical criterion of ± 1.65 SD (5th and 95th percentile of a normal distribution) is applied, the 'normal range' of birthweight would be from 1312 g to 2374 g.

On statistical criteria, therefore, a first-born boy at 32 weeks weighing 1400 g belongs to the same distribution as one weighing half as much again drawn from the same population. But that difference would quite rightly be seen as clinically significant. Although it is incumbent on researchers to test their research hypotheses, and statistical tests are frequently the most appropriate form of test, the clinician's practical interest may not be best served by the rigorous application of statistical criteria. The issue is taken up in chapter 9.

The concept of 'normal'

Standards are used clinically to assess whether the growth of a baby has departed from the 'normal'. 'Normal' is defined in terms of the sort of growth that might be expected if the pregnancy had followed the 'usual' pattern. For this reason 'unusual' pregnancies culminating, for example, in the birth of an anencephalic baby or twins are generally excluded in the derivation of standards for clinical use. The definition of 'unusual' is, of course, not axiomatic and the approach adopted in this work is discussed in detail in chapter 5.

The issue here, however, is that the concept of normal has different meanings for clinical and research purposes. For clinical purposes, the concept of 'normal' defines which cases should be included in the base population for the derivation of standards. For the researcher, the selection of cases for the base population depends on the focus of research.

ORGANISATION OF THE BOOK

Our work on this monograph started because we tried to understand the trends in birthweight over the last quarter of a century and encountered a number of puzzles which are described in chapter 2. Thereafter, the main body of the monograph is arranged in three sections: the first is the theoretical background, the second the empirical argument, and the third contains illustrations of the use of the standards in research. The first section consists of chapters 3, 4 and 5. Chapters 3 and 4 are the review chapters. Chapter 3 reviews the evidence about the relationship between those factors which are assumed to affect fetal growth and observed birthweight; and chapter 4 reviews a selection of recent surveys of birthweight focussing on their methodology. Chapter 5 draws together the reviews in the light of the theoretical literature in order first to classify the various factors which have been discussed in the literature, and second to propose a model of the relationship between the various factors which have been assumed to affect fetal growth and the resulting birthweight.

The second section consists of chapters 6, 7 and 8. Materials and statistical methods are discussed in chapter 6: material available in the Aberdeen Data Bank and the criteria for exclusion and inclusion are discussed first, followed by a brief overview of the methods to be used and the analytic strategy to be employed. Chapter 7 exemplifies the methods and the strategy with the Aberdeen data, by first exploring the correlation matrices and then investigating whether or not an appropriate functional form of the relationship between birthweight and gestation can be derived. Chapter 8 starts out from birthweight scores standardised for the gestational age, parity and the sex of the infant, and then estimates parameters for characteristics of the mother (her height, weight and age).

Chapters 9, 10 and 11, which constitute the third section of the book discuss and illustrate the possible uses of birthweight standards. Chapter 9 shows how these parameter estimates can be used to elaborate a set of standards for clinical practice, and discusses the errors that would be involved in using a normal approximation to the birthweight distributions.

Chapters 10 and 11 use the standards which have been developed to explore two particular issues in the literature and, in particular, the methodological difficulties involved. Chapter 10 looks at the problems of analysing the effects of social class upon birthweight, and chapter 11 considers the effect of smoking when its possible interaction with maternal weight and pre-eclampsia are taken into account.

The monograph concludes, in chapter 12 with a discussion of the implications for theory and practice of this analysis.

2
Birthweight trends since 1950

INTRODUCTION

This book is concerned with the derivation and exploitation of birthweight standards. In the chapters which follow, conceptual, methodological and technical problems in deriving and using birthweight standards are discussed in detail and at some length.

There is, however, a prior question of why such a detailed and lengthy treatment should be needed. Birthweight standards, such as those derived by Lubchenco *et al.* (1963) and Thomson *et al.* (1968) have been and are in widespread use both for clinical and research purposes, especially for the identification of a group of babies whose birthweight suggests that they have been growing at a considerably lower rate than is 'normal'. The 'growth retarded' group is usually defined as those babies falling below the 10th or 5th percentile of birthweight for gestation. In this context, Thomson (1983) has recently argued that:

> . . . any standard may be regarded as appropriate if the distributions *not necessarily the absolute values* of birthweight by gestation are reasonably similar to those of the population to be investigated.

The intention of this introductory chapter is, firstly, to show that, even within a particular locale (as it happens the same locale to that used by Thomson *et al.*, 1968) both the absolute values and the distributions of birthweight by gestation have changed over time. Secondly, we draw attention to some of the problems in discussing fetal growth rates on the basis of this kind of data and, in particular, the influence of changes in clinical practice and the changes in the distribution of 'abnormal' pregnancies over time. The implications of changes in the bivariate distribution of birthweight and gestation for the development of birthweight standards are discussed in the final section.

DATA

The data used in this chapter are drawn from the whole range of the Aberdeen Maternal and Neonatal Data Bank (Samphier and Thompson, 1982) which contains records of births in Aberdeen since 1948. The data presented relate to singleton live born babies whose mothers were resident in Aberdeen and where both gestation and last monthly period were 'certain'. Where appropriate, the data have been recoded to be compatible with the data used in the bulk of this monograph which are described in chapter 6. Particular recoding has included the conversion of birthweights originally coded in pounds and ounces (until 1976) to grammes and the week of gestation in which the birth occurred to 'completed weeks'. Note that the criterion of certainty and the estimate of length of gestation used in this chapter differ from those used in the rest of the book and discussed in chapter 6: the discrepancy arises from the need to ensure consistency over thirty years.

CHANGES IN THE BIRTHWEIGHT AND GESTATION

Changes in mean birthweight for gestation

In a recent article (Carr-Hill and Pritchard, 1983) we draw attention to the decline in mean birthweight for gestation in Aberdeen over the last thirty years. In particular, we commented upon the decline in mean birthweight for babies born before 37 weeks gestation ('pre-term'). The findings were not unique to Aberdeen (see Forbes and Smalls, 1983).

The pattern is shown in figure 2.1 which compares the mean birthweight for gestation in the early 1950s with the late 1970s; the data are reported in detail for each of the five year periods in table 2.1. With the exception of the 41st week of gestation, mean birthweight for each week of gestation was lower in the period 1976–1980 than in the period 1951–1956. For babies born between 32 and 36 weeks of gestation the average birthweight has fallen by a dramatic 350 grams between the two periods.

Intuitively, at least, this decline is rather surprising. On the general grounds that there has been a secular improvement in living standards over the last thirty years, it might have been expected that mean birthweight for gestation would have increased over the period. For example, stillbirth rates which, independently of improvements in late obstetric and early neonatal care, can be used as a broad indication of reproductive performance, have fallen sharply over the period; in Scotland from 26.9 per thousand in 1950 to 6.7 per thousand in 1980; and in Aberdeen from 17.0 per thousand to 6.3 per thousand. Note that the sharp change in stillbirth rates do not affect the overall distributions discussed in this chapter because the numbers involved are so small.

In spite of the pattern of declining birthweight at each gestation week and

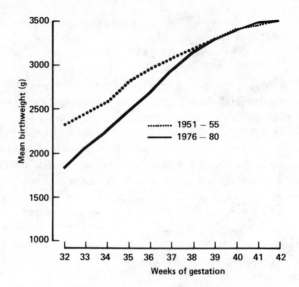

Figure 2.1 Mean birthweights by week of gestation, 1951-1955 and 1976-1980

Table 2.1 Mean and standard deviation of birthweight, numbers and cumulative distribution by gestation, proportions induced, primiparae and primiparae with proteinuric pre-eclampsia for gestational weeks 32–42 and mean maternal height in
the six five-year periods since 1950

(a) *1951-1955*

Weeks gestation	Mean birthweight	Standard deviation	N	Cumulative %	% induced	% prims	% prims PET
32	2319.5	654.4	45	0.4	6.7	46.7	19.0
33	2447.6	585.9	66	0.9	12.1	34.8	21.7
34	2592.2	559.2	114	1.8	6.3	39.5	6.7
35	2815.3	543.0	172	3.1	14.5	28.8	9.5
36	2959.3	501.7	344	5.8	15.7	40.2	16.5
Pre-term subtotal	2785.0	575.8	741	5.8	13.4	42.0	13.8
37	3069.8	452.6	663	11.0	16.6	40.7	10.0
38	3183.9	436.9	1558	23.2	15.0	39.8	8.1
39	3304.3	438.0	2960	46.4	12.8	39.3	6.4
40	3417.6	445.0	3773	76.0	14.7	41.6	3.8
41	3461.8	460.5	2261	93.8	25.7	42.4	1.9
42	3489.7	490.4	790	100.0	32.7	41.2	3.7
All gestations	3320.2	489.1	12746	100.0	17.4	40.9	5.4
Mean maternal height =	158.1						

Table 2.1 (*continued*)

(b) *1956–1960*

Weeks gestation	Mean birthweight	Standard deviation	N	Cumulative %	% induced	% prims	% prims PET
32	2098.4	684.0	39	0.3	12.8	48.7	10.5
33	2319.4	614.7	63	0.8	11.1	55.6	8.3
34	2566.7	593.6	83	1.4	15.7	50.6	19.0
35	2723.5	516.7	149	2.5	16.8	45.0	11.9
36	2912.1	498.7	302	4.7	12.9	44.0	10.5
Pre-term subtotal	2714.3	592.2	636	4.7	14.0	46.5	11.8
Weeks gestation							
37	3034.0	485.0	623	9.2	21.7	37.4	15.3
38	3167.9	449.7	1553	20.3	22.0	42.2	8.5
39	3304.2	435.8	3125	42.8	15.9	40.8	4.2
40	3424.8	440.1	4234	73.2	16.7	42.2	2.7
41	3494.8	453.1	2814	93.4	28.8	43.9	1.8
42	3497.3	473.6	937	100.0	48.8	42.0	1.3
All gestations	3338.2	491.4	13922	100.0	21.8	42.2	4.4
Mean maternal height =	158.3						

(c) *1961–1965*

Weeks gestation	Mean birthweight	Standard deviation	N	Cumulative %	% induced	% prims	% prims PET
32	1974.7	436.7	34	0.2	11.8	35.3	16.7
33	2264.1	561.2	69	0.7	21.7	50.7	20.0
34	2537.0	613.8	110	1.5	20.9	38.2	19.0
35	2746.1	569.4	184	2.8	21.7	37.4	7.5
36	2887.6	541.5	293	4.8	20.8	42.7	10.4
Pre-term subtotal	2686.6	612.2	690	4.8	17.2	40.7	12.5
Weeks gestation							
37	3024.5	483.4	665	9.4	25.4	39.2	10.0
38	3178.8	444.7	1758	21.6	27.7	38.4	7.6
39	3332.7	432.0	3309	44.6	18.9	38.7	2.9
40	3431.9	438.9	4349	74.7	21.2	40.4	2.4
41	3531.8	446.2	2740	93.7	29.7	41.1	1.6
42	3526.0	470.5	928	100.0	46.6	42.9	1.8
All gestations	3349.0	495.2	14459	100.0	24.9	40.4	3.7
Mean maternal height =	158.4						

Table 2.1 (*continued*)

(d) *1966-1970*

Weeks gestation	Mean birthweight	Standard deviation	N	Cumulative %	% induced	% prims	% prims PET
32	1908.2	396.7	49	0.4	16.3	42.9	28.6
33	2175.1	536.1	70	0.9	20.0	45.7	18.8
34	2402.8	474.1	82	1.5	22.0	51.2	11.9
35	2632.9	475.5	168	2.8	22.6	41.7	10.0
36	2813.3	517.0	261	4.8	26.1	46.4	10.7
Pre-term subtotal	2570.4	569.0	630	4.8	23.2	46.3	12.9
Weeks gestation							
37	2996.4	482.7	592	9.3	31.8	38.3	14.5
38	3145.0	446.9	1576	21.3	37.9	40.2	11.4
39	3305.9	442.4	3042	44.5	32.8	40.0	4.4
40	3399.2	426.5	4165	76.2	38.8	41.4	1.7
41	3474.4	445.6	2535	95.5	49.5	41.6	1.3
42	3461.4	453.9	583	100.0	67.8	44.3	1.2
All gestations	3306.4	493.2	13123	100.0	39.6	41.2	4.5

Mean maternal height = 158.8

(e) *1971-1975*

Weeks gestation	Mean birthweight	Standard deviation	N	Cumulative %	% induced	% prims	% prims PET
32	1983.2	520.0	28	0.3	32.1	85.7	20.5
33	2102.7	381.5	33	0.6	21.2	44.5	6.7
34	2400.5	425.0	73	1.3	24.7	49.3	22.2
35	2541.6	537.1	103	2.3	26.2	51.5	13.2
36	2835.2	462.1	220	4.3	25.5	45.0	9.1
Pre-term subtotal	2594.5	544.9	457	4.3	25.6	49.7	13.2
Weeks gestation							
37	2986.9	466.7	441	8.4	33.7	45.4	12.0
38	3165.6	433.3	1084	18.5	34.3	43.3	12.4
39	3312.6	433.7	2380	40.6	36.5	42.2	8.9
40	3427.4	425.8	3423	72.4	42.5	43.1	4.1
41	3499.9	445.4	2528	95.9	58.6	45.0	4.4
42	3412.9	421.6	460	100.0	71.1	43.6	4.1
All gestations	3338.7	483.9	10773	100.0	44.3	43.9	6.8

Mean maternal height = 159.4

Table 2.1 *(continued)*

(f) *1976-1980*

Weeks gestation	Mean birthweight	Standard deviation	N	Cumulative %	% induced	% prims	% prims PET
32	1818.8	283.3	24	0.3	25.0	45.8	18.2
33	2065.0	319.4	36	0.7	22.2	44.4	12.5
34	2251.9	406.2	52	1.3	26.9	44.2	34.8
35	2479.7	428.2	86	2.3	29.1	51.2	20.5
36	2671.3	403.7	143	4.0	31.5	51.7	20.3
Pre-term subtotal	2435.0	474.3	341	4.0	28.7	49.3	21.4
Weeks gestation							
37	2939.3	472.3	321	7.9	23.8	41.1	16.7
38	3150.9	415.6	812	17.8	30.9	43.2	14.9
39	3306.2	437.5	1951	41.5	32.8	42.6	7.8
40	3392.9	423.3	2667	73.9	37.8	43.1	4.1
41	3488.1	408.7	1840	96.3	52.3	44.8	5.7
42	3498.6	443.9	295	100.0	67.1	44.4	3.1
All gestations	3316.1	482.7	8227	100.0	39.3	43.3	7.6
Mean maternal height =	159.4						

particularly the sharp differences at early gestational ages, the overall mean birthweight for babies born between 32 and 42 weeks gestation has remained relatively consistent, showing only a slight decrease between the early 1950s (mean birthweight 3320.2 g) and the period 1976-1980 (mean birthweight 3316.1 g). Clearly, there has to have been a shift in the distribution of gestational ages in order to account for this apparent anomaly. Moreover, the differences in the graphs of mean birthweight for gestation have interesting implications for the discussion of changes over these thirty years.

One could interpret the graphs in figure 2.1 as suggesting that the rate of fetal growth between week 32 and week 38 has become much faster over the last thirty years; if this were so then the need for new birthweight standards is axiomatic. An alternative view is that, irrespective of the distribution of gestational ages, the distribution of 'normal' birthweights at each gestational age has not changed but that, for a variety of reasons, there are more growth retarded babies born alive at the earlier weeks. The implications of this view is that commonly used standards, whilst they would identify a higher proportion of growth retarded babies, remain appropriate. A third view is that there has been a fundamental shift in the distribution of gestational ages which has implications for the distribution of birthweights following both 'normal' and 'abnormal' pregnancies: for an elaboration of this view, see below. *A priori*, the latter view is more complex and the analyses in the remaining sections of this chapter therefore concentrate on the problems it poses.

Changes in the distribution of gestational ages

The detail of the changes in the distribution of gestational ages is shown in table 2.1. Figure 2.2 compares the cumulative distribution of gestational ages

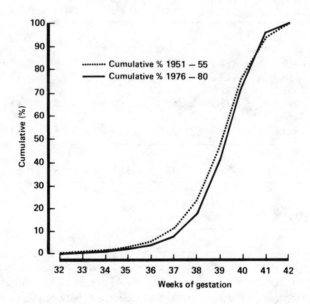

Figure 2.2   Cumulative distribution of gestational ages, 1951–1955 and 1976–1980

for the period 1951–1955 with that for the period 1976–1980. The cumulative distributions are significantly different (Kolmogorov-Smirnov test KS_{max} = 0.065 at 38 weeks $p < 0.001$).

The principal change has been that births in the more recent period tended to be more concentrated into weeks 39, 40 and 41 than was the case in the period 1951-1956. There has been a progressive decline in the proportion of births occurring at each gestational week up to and including the 38th week. The proportion of births occurring in week 42 has declined steadily, but with a sharp fall in the late 1960s.

A possible interpretation

In order to account for *both* the trend towards later gestational ages *and* the pattern of declining birthweight for gestation, especially at the earlier gestational ages, one could tentatively advance the following hypothesis. Such a hypothesis relies on the dual notion that:

(1) the 'natural' length of a pregnancy is somewhere around 39/40 weeks so that pregnancies which end in a birth in the earlier weeks of gestation are, in some ways, 'abnormal'; and

(2) that for a woman with given characteristics, the fetal growth process is a physiological invariant across time.

It is important to emphasise that this latter notion refers only to an individual woman. In examining the aggregate distributions of birthweight and of gestation, secular changes in the overall distribution of maternal or pregnancy characteristics which might affect the fetal growth rate become important. More specifically, in the development of standards of birthweight for gestation, the issue is whether or not there have been any secular changes which might affect the fetal growth rate for a given sex and parity.

Whilst there have, of course, been shifts in the incidence of several characteristics which have been suggested in the literature as likely to affect the fetal growth rate (see the next two chapters), the only obvious candidates which might have affected the whole birthweight distribution are maternal size and smoking habits. Unfortunately, the data are not available to examine secular changes in maternal pre-pregnancy weight or smoking habits, but we can explore the possibility of a trend in maternal height. The mean maternal heights are given in table 2.1 and it can be seen that, although they have increased slightly, there has been no significant change.

If, on the other hand, the secular changes in living conditions and the improvements in antenatal care have affected, not the rate of fetal growth but the factors that determine the length of gestation, then the average birthweights at the main gestational ages (39, 40 and 41 weeks) would have remained relatively constant over time although the proportions of births occurring in those weeks would have increased.

The implication of this argument is that, as the fraction of births occurring in the earlier weeks of gestation decreases, the babies born in those weeks would increasingly represent the outcome of pregnancies unaffected by the improvement in living conditions and/or of pregnancies where the 'abnormality' has proved, thus far, to be intractible to the improvements in antenatal care. If we further assume that these 'abnormalities' are associated, in general, with a lower fetal growth rate, the effect would be a marked lowering in average birthweight for those weeks.

It might be claimed, on the basis of the decline in stillbirth rates (see above), that improvements in antenatal care and obstetric management have contributed to the proportion of live births following 'abnormal pregnancies' through the improved survival of affected fetuses. But the number of such 'additional', possibly lighter babies, is at most 20 per thousand in the recent epoch (based on the observed differences in stillbirth rates) and the overall effect on mean birthweight and patterns of gestation can only, therefore, be minimal.

Unfortunately, although such an account would explain the pattern of declining birthweight for gestation, there is no way of testing it in detail with the data available. The changes have, of course, been more complex than such an account would suggest and three specific shifts are examined below.

Firstly, we examine the tendency towards the more active management of 'abnormal' pregnancies especially through induction; secondly, we look at the changing balance between primiparae and multiparae, and finally, we explore the implications of shifts in the diagnosed incidence of pre-eclampsia (which is the most common pregnancy-related disorder which affects birthweight).

The argument in all three cases turns upon a comparison between the early 1950s and the late 1970s of the relative incidence of the phenomenon at each week of gestation (see figures 2.3, 2.6 and 2.8) and upon the mean birthweight at the pre-term weeks when the changes in mean birthweight have been greatest (see figures 2.5, 2.7 and 2.9). The section on induction includes some additional material because of the complexity of that argument.

CHANGES IN THE CHARACTERISTICS OF PREGNANCIES

Changes in induction practice

Across the six five-yearly periods since 1950, the rate of induction has increased from 17.4% in the early 1950s to 44.3% in the early 1970s, falling back to 39.3% in the most recent period (see table 2.1). There was a sharp increase in the proportion of induced labours during the 1960s when the induction rate increased from 24.9% in the early 1960s to 39.6% in the period 1966-1970. Figure 2.3 shows the rate of induction by week of gestation for the first and last periods. With the exception of the 37th week, induction rates have more than doubled for each week of gestation, representing a substantial change in this aspect of obstetric management.

The effect of induction, of course, is that 'induced babies' are born earlier than would have been the case had the pregnancy been allowed to continue until a spontaneous onset of labour. The effect of increasing the proportion of inductions ought to have been *ceteris paribus* an overall tendency for gestations to be shorter. Indeed, this may account for the reduction in the proportion of births at 42 weeks, which coincides with the sharp increase in the induction rate in the 1960s. However, with this single exception of 42 weeks gestation, the increase in the induction rate is running counter to the trend towards longer gestations commented upon above.

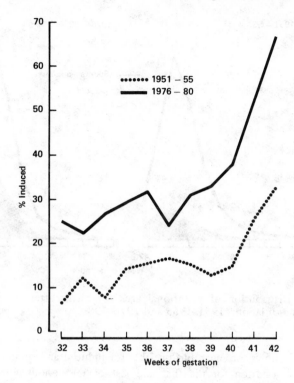

Figure 2.3   Percentage of labours induced by week of gestation, 1951–1955 and 1976–1980

Figure 2.4 (see over) shows the distribution of gestational ages for the periods 1951-55 and 1976-80 with the proportions of induced births shaded. In both periods the rate of induction was less in the 'pre-term' weeks than among the later gestations. The numbers involved in the pre-term weeks are relatively small: thus 99 (0.78% of all births between 32 and 42 weeks) were induced pre-term in the early 1950s whilst the corresponding figure for the most recent period was 98 (1.19%). The effect of the increased proportion of inductions in these early weeks on the whole distribution of gestational ages must therefore be marginal.

While the effects of the increased proportion of inductions are probably not great on the overall distribution of gestational ages, their effects on the distribution of birthweight for gestation may still be large at particular weeks. The decision to induce represents a clinical judgement about the progress of the pregnancy in which, in the earlier gestational weeks, the risks of pre-term delivery are weighed against the risks of continuing the pregnancy. The decision to induce is often related to a diagnosed abnormality in the apparent growth of the fetus, and changes in pre-term induction rates may be one mechanism by which less well grown babies are differentially born in the earlier weeks.

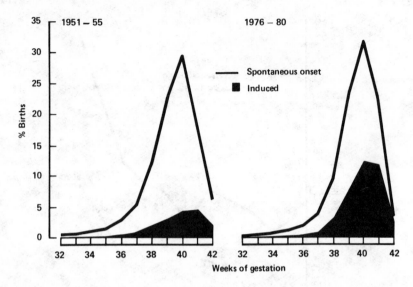

Figure 2.4 Distribution of gestational ages for births after spontaneous and induced onset of labour, 1951–1955 and 1976–1980

Figure 2.5 shows the mean birthweights for induced and spontaneous births by weeks of gestation for the first and last of the periods considered. The detailed figures are presented in table 2.1.

Overall, across all gestations, induced babies were lighter than babies delivered after spontaneous onset of labour in the 1950s and 1960s and heavier in the 1970s. Whilst, in both the earlier and later periods, there is hardly any difference between induced and spontaneous labours among babies delivered at the peak term weeks (38, 39 and 40 weeks), there are interesting variations at other gestational ages.

Thus, whilst in the earlier periods babies delivered after spontaneous labours at 41 and 42 weeks were substantially heavier than those induced (by about 90 grammes), no such difference appears in the later period. Moreover, a much higher proportion of those delivering at 41 and 42 weeks were induced in the later period and inspection of the reasons given for induction shows that most inductions at those weeks were for non-medical reasons.

More importantly, whilst in both the earlier and later periods, those delivered after spontaneous onset of labours were heavier than those induced, the differences were considerably larger in the early 1950s (see figure 2.5). As can be seen from the diagram, this arises essentially from the much larger mean birthweights of those delivered after spontaneous onset of labour in the earlier period. In fact, those delivered after spontaneous onset of labours in the later period have similar mean birthweights to those who have been induced in either period.

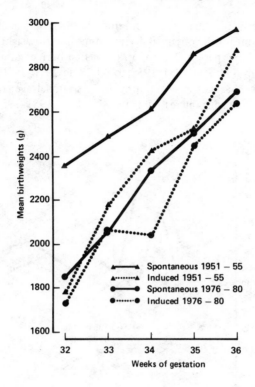

Figure 2.5 Mean birthweights following spontaneous and induced onset of labour, pre-term births, 1951–1955 and 1976–1980

These observations do not sit happily with our earlier suggestion that the increasing proportion of inductions at the pre-term weeks reflected an increasing concentration of 'abnormal' pregnancies among those delivering pre-term. Indeed, these observations suggest the rather simpler view that, irrespective of how the labour started, pre-term deliveries have become progressively an out-come of abnormal pregnancies. In a complementary fashion, those whose labour started spontaneously pre-term in the earlier period would now, given the secular changes which have been hypothesised to promote longer gestations, tend to start labour later and, therefore, would be beyond the range included in this figure.

Parity

One of the features of changes in the pattern of fertility over the last thirty years has been the trend towards smaller families (for Scotland, see Pritchard and Thompson, 1982). This trend is reflected in obstetric data by an increase in the proportion of first born children as a percentage of all births. Since first born babies tend to be lighter than later born, shifts in the proportions of primiparae may help to account for the observed decline in mean birthweight overall.

Over the thirty year period, the proportion of first born children has increased in Aberdeen, from 40.9% in 1951-1955 to 43.3% in 1976-1980. As figure 2.6 shows this change has not been uniform by gestational age; the proportions delivering pre-term having increased from 42.1% in 1951-1955 to 49.3% in 1976-1980.

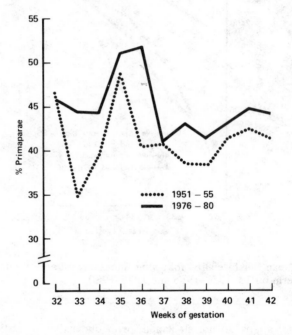

Figure 2.6 Deliveries to primiparae as a percentage of all births by week of gestation, 1951-1955 and 1976-1980

Although such marginal shifts are unlikely to have had any great impact on mean birthweight by gestation, it is of interest to compare the birthweights of first and later born amongst the pre-term groups in the two periods. As figure 2.7 shows, in the earlier period, the mean birthweight of later born pre-term babies was consistently higher than that of first born pre-term babies by a considerable amount (over 200 grams at each gestational week). This is in marked contrast to the pattern in the later period, where the difference between first and later born is relatively small, the maximum difference being 180 grams at 34 weeks which is a notable exception to the small differences at the other pre-term gestational weeks.

More interesting is the fact that, in these pre-term weeks, primiparae in the earlier period are substantially heavier than even multiparae in the later period at every pre-term gestational age. Note that this is not true for term weeks.

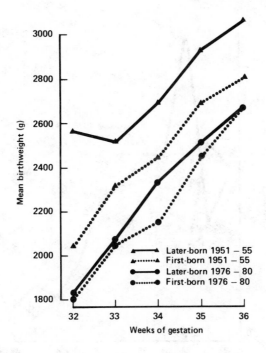

Figure 2.7   Mean birthweights for first- and later-born babies by week of gestation, pre-term births, 1951–1955 and 1976–1980

These observations do not support an account of the dramatic decline in
mean birthweight in the pre-term weeks. For, although there has been an increasing proportion of primiparae, the mean birthweights of primiparae then were
heavier than the mean birthweight of all babies now, irrespective of parity. Once
again, however, these observations are consistent with the view that a pre-term
delivery in the recent period is more 'abnormal' than it was in the earlier period.

Pre-eclampsia

This section considers only primiparae as the incidence of pre-eclampsia among
multiparae is much lower (2.0% compared to 7.6% in 1976-1980). The pattern
of incidence of proteinuric pre-eclampsia has changed over the thirty years. The
shift shown in figure 2.8 may, of course, be the result of improved antenatal
care and consequently of a higher rate of detection of these pathological cases.
Indeed, given the known changes in the pattern of antenatal care, irrespective of
any real trend over the intervening years, we clearly have to be cautious about
interpreting this shift in terms of a change in the incidence of the disorder.
Nevertheless, it does look as if the proportions of pre-term labour where the
woman developed proteinuric pre-eclampsia has increased (from 13.8% in the
earlier period to 21.4% in the later period). At the same time, in both earlier and

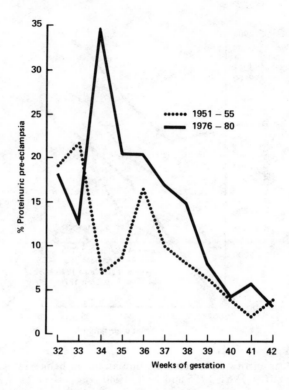

Figure 2.8   Incidence (%) of proteinuric pre-eclampsia amongst primiparae by week of gestation at delivery, 1951–1955 and 1976–1980

later periods, cases of proteinuric pre-eclampsia are concentrated in the pre-term weeks (*c.* 13% of cases in both periods as compared to around 5% of all births).

The comparison of mean birthweight for gestational weeks between the normotensive and proteinuric groups in the first and last periods is presented in figure 2.9. In both periods babies born to normotensive mothers are usually substantially heavier than those born to proteinuric mothers. More importantly, there has been an overall downward shift in mean birthweight for gestation separately for the normotensive and proteinuric groups.

Given the numbers involved (see table 2.1) the mean birthweights of the proteinuric groups are similar in both periods, so that the fact that the incidence of proteinuric pre-eclampsia has increased cannot account for the shift in mean birthweights. On the other hand, there clearly has been an increase in abnormal pregnancies (in this case, those with proteinuric pre-eclampsia) and the decline in mean birthweight of babies born to normotensive mothers is, once again, consistent with the view that a pre-term delivery in the recent period is more 'abnormal' than it was in the earlier period.

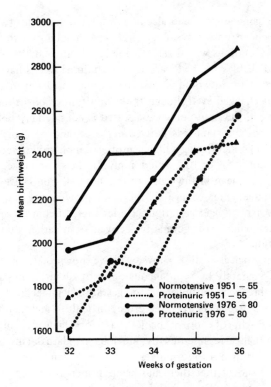

Figure 2.9 Mean birthweights in normative and proteinuric pre-eclamptic pregnancies by week of gestation, 1951–1955 and 1976–1980

SUMMARY AND DISCUSSION

This chapter was not intended to offer an explanation of the changes that have happened in mean birthweight for gestation over a thirty-year period. Such an explanation would entail a detailed epidemiological study. Rather, it was intended to present and explore those changes with a view to considering their implications for the development of birthweight standards. Certainly, the changes have been considerable and may be gauged by the fact that the mean birthweight for later born babies at 36 weeks in the period 1976–1980 was just below the 32nd percentile in Thomson *et al.*'s (1968) standards: indeed, 25.1% of such babies would fall below the 10th centile and 13.6% below the 5th centile.

Clearly, it would be possible to argue that secular changes in living conditions have affected the pattern of fetal growth in such a way that it is slower during early pregnancy and faster during, say, the last trimester than was the case in previous periods. *Prima facie*, this is what figure 2.1 says, and none of the material presented in this chapter can refute that view. Of course, in this case, the need for new birthweight standards is axiomatic.

However, the same graph could also be interpreted in at least two other ways which do not depend on a physiological change in fetal growth rate. Both of these other interpretations would rely on the argument that the proportions of 'growth retarded' babies born at particular gestational weeks have changed. In the first case the argument would be that the 'normal' birthweight at a particular gestation has not changed even though the proportion of births on the basis of which a 'normal' birthweight could be assessed is considerably reduced. Under these circumstances the standards derived earlier would probably be the most appropriate, although identifying a higher proportion of 'growth retarded' babies than the conventional 5% or 10% would imply. In the second case, however, the inference is that the mean birthweights of the 'normal' group have reduced: not because of a fundamental change in the fetal growth rate but because the mothers tend to have longer gestations. Under these circumstances, the appropriateness of the standard of 'normality' derived from earlier studies would be called into question.

In the epidemiological analysis above, we have shown that, for three 'normal' groups, defined separately by spontaneous onset of labour, multiparity or being normotensive – the mean birthweight for gestation has declined substantially over the last twenty-five years. It is, therefore, difficult to maintain the view that the mean birthweight of normal babies has not changed, which calls into question the normality represented by previous standards. This is one of the main reasons for setting out to formulate a new set of standards.

We have, also, shown that there has been an increase in the proportions of births following 'abnormal' pregnancies in the pre-term weeks. In particular, induction differentially selects such babies, and proteinuric pre-eclampsia is associated with reduced fetal growth. Changes of this sort, in their own right, have important implications for the derivation of birthweight standards. If the proportion of 'growth retarded' babies varies with gestation at all, let alone in the systematic way suggested by the pattern of changes in mean birthweight for gestation shown above, then the meaning of a diagnostic criterion based on a fixed proportion of birthweight distribution at individual gestational weeks is far from clear.

Furthermore, as we shall discuss at some length in chapters 5 and 6, the estimation of fetal growth from a sequence of mean birthweights would be impossible. The increment in mean birthweight between two consecutive weeks of gestation would represent not only the fetal growth that would 'normally' occur between those gestational ages, but also the relative proportions of those with 'abnormal' fetal growth who happened to be born at those weeks. We cannot know these latter proportions by reference to the distributions of birthweight, whether in current or previous data. It would, therefore, be very courageous indeed to suggest that earlier standards such as those of Thomson *et al.* would be in any sense 'more appropriate' for a current population than standards based on more recent distributions. Indeed, the use of smoothing procedures on the basis of an assumed relationship between the pattern of a sequence of birthweights and a notional smooth process of fetal growth would be particularly dubious.

In more detail, this chapter firstly considered the role of induction in the changes in mean birthweight for gestation. It was suggested that induction might change both the distribution of gestational ages and the distribution of birthweights at particular gestational weeks. While the former suggestion is axiomatically true, investigation of the suggestion that the distribution of birthweights at particular gestational ages might have been affected by the changes in induction practice appears not to be true in the most recent period. In 1976–1980, babies born after labour was induced had similar birthweights to the group who were born after a spontaneous onset of labour.

The changes in the distribution of gestational ages brought about by the increased induction rate do, however, cause particular difficulties for the derivation of birthweight standards. These difficulties are discussed in detail in chapter 5. Since the distribution of gestational ages is affected not only by biological processes but, differentially, by clinical practice, the significance of being born at a particular gestational age becomes problematic.

Secondly, the effects of changes in the distributions of parity were considered. Had the effects of these changing distributions accounted for some of the changes that had taken place over the thirty years, it could have been argued that standards controlling for parity would remain appropriate. However, although the distribution of parities has changed, in particular gestational weeks, this change did not offer an explanation of the changes in mean birthweight for gestation.

Finally, we considered whether the incidence of pre-eclampsia might account for at least some part of the changes. Although the increased incidence of proteinuric pre-eclampsia did not substantively help to account for the changes, it does provide a specific illustration of the difficulty of the concept of 'normality' birthweight standards. We have shown above how different incidences of pre-eclampsia in different gestational weeks may affect the value of statistical diagnostic criteria for growth retardation. Furthermore, an overall increase in the incidence, which may be mediated to an unknown extent by improved diagnosis of the disease, casts some doubt on the appropriateness of the use of standards derived at different times or elsewhere. The whole question of whether standards ought to incorporate estimates of the effects of 'non-normal' factors, such as those associated with pregnancy-related disorders, is addressed in chapter 5.

Overall, then, the argument of this chapter has been that the distributions of birthweight for gestation have changed over the last twenty-five years in Aberdeen. Not only have the distributions of birthweight at particular gestational weeks changed, but also the distribution of gestational ages has changed and the association of birthweight and gestation has changed. These changes mean that the relationship between standards derived in an earlier period and the observed distributions in the most recent period has changed in ways that are by no means simple or obvious. The general lesson we wish to draw from these changes is that standards derived from the empirical observation of distributions of birthweight only directly relate to the sample observed. The use of standards derived at a particular time in a particular location at other times and other locations is problematic because the meanings of those standards for other samples is unclear.

As the rest of this book shows, the derivation of standards for a particular sample is both a conceptually and statistically complex task. In resolving these complexities, however, it becomes possible to derive standards with unequivocal meanings for *research* use. However, Thomson's (1983) comment on the *clinical* value of standards also applies to the standards we derive:

> The standard itself is no more than a statistical reference grid and centiles should not be interpreted as implying different levels of risk in themselves unless there is external evidence showing that such differential risks do in fact exist.

SECTION 2

Theoretical Background

The three chapters in this section form the theoretical background for the development of birthweight standards. Chapters 3 and 4 are reviews of the literature on factors affecting birthweight and on birthweight surveys and constitute the knowledge base for the theoretical models discussed in chapter 5.

3

Factors affecting birthweight

INTRODUCTION

This chapter is concerned to review, principally from epidemiological evidence, major variables whose influence on birthweight has been documented and discussed and which might play a part in a birthweight survey. Of course, birthweight depends on the number and size of cells present in the neonate. Ultimately, too, it may be that the various influences on birthweight discussed here and elsewhere will find their explanation at the level of cellular processes (cf. Dobbing and Sands, 1978); but this is not the level of explanation in this monograph. The review of the literature is by no means exhaustive, but is intended to inform and establish a basis for the analyses which follow. Nor is it intended to be especially original: it draws heavily on Hytten and Leitch (1971). To some extent, therefore, the contents of this chapter reflect the issues addressed later in this book and is shaped by data routinely collected in Aberdeen.

REVIEW OF FACTORS AFFECTING BIRTHWEIGHT

Gestation

It is universally accepted that mean birthweight increases with increasing gestational age, although the relationship between gestation and birthweight is commonly reported as non-linear, especially beyond 42 weeks gestation (Karn and Penrose, 1951; Love and Kinch, 1965). The measurement of gestation and its relationship to birthweight forms the focus of much of the analysis and discussion which follows and for this reason it is noted here mainly for the sake of completeness (see especially chapters 5, 7 and 12). In general, of all the factors considered, gestation represents the most important, of itself accounting for over a fifth of the statistical variance in birthweight.

It is, however, of some importance to note that the estimation of gestational age is by no means precise. The date of conception is rarely known and estimates are nearly always based on the first day of the last menstrual period. Data on the date of the last menstrual period are, themselves, notoriously unreliable (Neligan, 1965) and the widespread use of the contraceptive pill adds a further element of uncertainty in some cases (Chamberlain, 1975).

Although it is generally agreed that ovulation occurs about 14 days before the expected first day of the *next* menstrual period, Birkbeck *et al.* (1975) adduce evidence to suggest that ovulation may vary by up to a week relative to the expected start of the next menstrual period. Further, while there is an assumption that fertilisation takes place shortly after ovulation the actual interval between ovulation and fertilisation is itself likely to vary. Therefore, even with careful recording and coding of data about the last menstrual period (and the usual menstrual cycle) uncertainties about the intervals from the date of the beginning of the last menstrual period to ovulation and from ovulation to conception will remain.

To these uncertainties must be added the variation introduced by expressing gestation in terms of 'completed weeks'. For example, '40 completed weeks' means not less than 280 days and not more than 286 days. Altogether, the usual citation of a specific length of gestation in weeks should more properly be referred to as a range of $\pm 1\frac{1}{2}$ weeks around the nominal gestation.

Genetic factors

Attempts to define the influences of the contribution of genetic factors on birth-weight are complicated by the effects of the 'environment' the mother provides for the growing fetus. In a set of classic animal experiments, Walton and Hammond (1938) made reciprocal crosses between Shetland ponies and Shire horses, the latter being four times the weight of the former. In either cross, the birthweights of the cross-bred foals were similar to those of maternal pure-bred foals. Joubert and Hammond (1954) performed a similar set of experiments using South Devon and Dexter cattle. Calves born to Dexter cows inseminated by South Devon cows were slightly larger than the pure-bred Dexter calves and much smaller than the pure-bred South Devon calves.

In humans, Morton (1955) showed a positive correlation between the birth-weights of half-siblings with different fathers and no such correlation between the birthweights of half-siblings with different mothers. Robson (1955) found correlations between the birthweights of maternal first cousins but not between the birthweights of paternal first cousins. More recently, Pritchard *et al.* (1983) have reported an association between birthweight and paternal stature. In view of the controversy surrounding the effects of recombination or heterosis within a given population (*vide*, for example, Morton *et al.*, 1967) the nature of the genetic component in birthweight may be more relevant to birthweight surveys than is immediately apparent, and is discussed further in chapter 12. In general, however, we would concur with Roberts' (1976) comment that the knowledge of the inheritance of birthweight is far from satisfactory.

Under the broad heading of genetic factors, it is convenient to include a mention of the effects of congenital anomalies. Brent and Jensch (1967) showed that a variety of autosomal anomalies are associated with small for gestational age babies. In the case of some other conditions, not uniquely associated with gross chromosomal abnormality, such as anencephaly (Usher and Maclean, 1974) or cardiovascular malformation (Levy *et al.*, 1978), the associated growth retardation may be the result of both genetic change and abnormal fetal function.

Sex of infant

Male babies tend to be heavier than female babies of the same gestation. This finding appears consistently in a wide variety of different populations from Australian aborigines (Kettle, 1960) to Aberdonians (Thomson *et al.*, 1968), from Canadians (Love and Kinch, 1965) to Maltese (Camilleri and Cremona, 1970). Although variations do occur (Adams and Niswander, 1968), in general the reported difference is betweeen 120 and 150 g.

There is some debate about the gestational age at which sex differences in fetal weight become apparent. Thomson *et al.* (1968) found no difference prior to 32 or 33 weeks gestation while Lubchenco *et al.* (1963) found a difference as early as 24 weeks. Milner and Richards (1974) showed an effect of sex on birthweight from 28 weeks increasing to term. All surveys are hampered by small numbers at early gestation. Sex differences in birthweight in early gestations are demonstrated in relation to recent Aberdeen data in later analyses (see chapters 7, 8 and 12).

Parity

The positive association between birthweight and increasing parity has also been widely and consistently reported. Primigravidae are more likely to give birth to babies small for gestational age (McDonald, 1962; Scott and Usher, 1966) and multigravidae are more likely to give birth to excessively large babies (Bolton, 1959; McEwan and Murdoch, 1966).

Although there is general agreement about a positive correlation, the agreement extends only to the differences between babies of primigravidae and multigravidae. While Thomson *et al.* (1968) report no further increase after the second pregnancy, Camilleri and Cremona (1970) in Malta and Mills and Seng (1954) in Singapore found that birthweight increases up to the ninth or tenth pregnancy. It may be that the association between high parity and adverse socio-economic circumstances in Aberdeen is not so marked in Malta and Singapore. Billewicz and Thomson (1973) indicate that career-wise analysis shows increasing birthweight over a woman's fertility history, although they argue that it is related to increasing maternal weight. Although her analysis is flawed, Dowding's (1981) study suggests that birth order effects in birthweight surveys may be accounted for in socio-economic terms. An analysis of Aberdeen data is presented in chapter 8 of this book and the issue is considered further in chapter 12.

Maternal age

The majority of post-war publications conclude that when the effect of maternal age is examined controlling for parity, it has little effect. However, carefully documented exceptions do exist in the literature. Karn and Penrose (1951), Fraccaro (1955) and Selvin and Janerich (1971) all conclude that birthweight increases with maternal age until the age of about 30 with a slight tendency to decline thereafter.

Although Scott and Usher (1966) report no age trend in mothers giving birth to babies small for gestational age, both Selvin and Janerich (1971) and Miller *et al.* (1977, 1978) argue that teenage pregnancy is associated with small babies. The latter authors also suggest that women over the age of 35 have a higher risk of bearing children small for gestational age, although Grimes and Gross (1981) did not find this in their analysis of births to black women in Atlanta.

Maternal size

In most species, including humans, there is a positive relationship between maternal size and birthweight (Leitch *et al.*, 1959). Maternal size itself may reflect genetic characteristics but may also be determined by environmental or disease factors during childhood. In turn, the effects of maternal size on birthweight may be genetic, but may also relate to the environment the mother provides for the growing fetus (see the discussion in chapter 5).

The two most frequently measured parameters of maternal size are height and weight. Billewicz *et al.* (1962) showed that height is uncorrelated with an index of weight-for-height and Thomson *et al.* (1968) have argued that the effects of height and weight-for-height on birthweight may be considered independently. This argument is commented upon later but, in the context of the review in this chapter, effects of height and weight are considered separately.

Maternal height

The positive correlation between maternal height and birthweight is a universal finding. Thomson *et al.* (1968), for example, showed a difference of 200–300 g between the shortest women in their survey (less than 5 ft 1 in) and the tallest (more than 5 ft 4 in). This difference was similar among women who were underweight, of average weight, and overweight.

Thomson (1971) further showed that, when birthweight was plotted against maternal height for a number of different populations with different mean birthweights, the slopes of the graphs were approximately parallel. This finding would argue that maternal height of itself has a comparable effect on birthweight in different populations.

Maternal weight

Maternal weight is, of course, related to maternal height. If the relative effects of 'thin-ness' and 'fat-ness' (in terms of deviation from 'normal size') are to be considered some index of adiposity provides a better parameter than gross weight. Using weight/height ratios, Love and Kinch (1965) found a positive correlation between maternal weight-for-height and birthweight. Several studies (Tompkins *et al.*, 1955; Miller *et al.*, 1977, 1978) have shown that being underweight is a significant maternal risk factor associated with babies small for gestational age. Luke and Petrie (1980) found, at the other extreme, that among overweight women, increasing weight had a detrimental effect on birthweight. The effect of the mother being very underweight is further commented upon in the discussion of maternal nutrition (below). The high incidence of abnormal glucose tolerance among obese women, noted by Sutherland *et al.* (1970) and its association with excessively large babies is discussed in the review of the effects of maternal disease on birthweight under the heading 'diabetes'.

Ethnic origin

Meredith (1970) has gathered data from 230 sources summarising the data into 78 major national or ethnic groups. Mean birthweights vary widely from 2400 g for a New Guinea tribe to 3600 g for Amerindians. Roberts (1976) derived averages for broader ethnic groups, showing a difference of just over 500 g between Indian and 'caucasoid' mean birthweights. Dawson *et al.* (1982) have shown differences in perinatal outcomes for low birthweight (under 2500 g) babies born to white European and Punjabi mothers in Hillingdon and argued that the application of 'caucasian' birthweight standards to all ethnic groups should be abandoned.

In spite of all the widely reported differences in mean birthweight between different ethnic groups, disparities in many of the other factors which of themselves influence birthweight confound the results of such surveys. Maternal size, for example, may be related to ethnic origin, but also to maternal nutrition both during childhood and pregnancy. Different patterns of maternal disease or of antenatal and obstetric care may play their parts in the observed differences. A variety of studies (e.g. Goldstein, 1947; Hendricks, 1967; Grundy *et al.*, 1978; Sibert *et al.*, 1978) show wide differences within ethnic groups dependent upon the presence or absence of adverse factors, and Barron (1983) has reviewed recent work and suggested the need for more precise data before the role of ethnicity can be clarified.

Maternal nutrition

The effects of extreme maternal malnutrition on birthweight have been documented (e.g. Antonov, 1947; Smith, 1947). Thus, Campbell and MacGillivray (1975) showed that 'severe' dietary restriction (1200 calorie diet) in the last trimester of pregnancy caused a reduction in birthweight. Although Rush *et al.* (1980) failed to show an improvement brought about by nutritional supplementation, Stein and Susser (1975) had already shown that the effects of maternal nutrition on birthweight were negligible over a threshold of about 1700 calories.

It is beyond the scope of this review to delve deeper into the process over which maternal malnutrition affects birthweight. Thomson (1957) has discussed the problems of analysis at some length and mentions difficulties of measurement, interpretation and the multifactorial nature of nutritional differences. The problems and current findings were debated at some length at the Workshop on Nutrition of the Child (1981) on maternal nutritional status and fetal outcome and it may be that, in overcoming these difficulties, the controversy will be resolved and it will become possible to assess the influence of various parameters of maternal nutrition on birthweight. Thomson's (1957) summary, however, still seems relevant:

> ...We are thus faced with a dilemma: on the one hand, a not unreasonable belief backed by much cogent evidence that the nutrition of women must be important, and on the other hand, the failure of survey methods to prove that this is so.

Maternal disease

It is beyond the scope of this review to detail all the diseases which a woman may suffer from or acquire during her pregnancy which may affect the birthweight of her baby. Brent and Jensch (1967) examined a large number of publications dealing with maternal disease during pregnancy and found that, where birthweight data were available, analysis was complicated by the difficulty of separating the effects of disease from those of treatment. A variety of maternal infections have been associated with growth retardation (Stevenson, 1977). Some, like rubella, involve the infection of the fetus *in utero* (e.g. Hardy, 1969), others, like malaria, usually do not involve congenital infection (e.g. Jeliffe, 1968). Bishop (1964) found a reduction in birthweight for gestation in women with a small heart volume, and congenital heart disease has been shown to have an adverse effect on birthweight (Batson, 1974). Two conditions, hypertension and diabetes, have been the focus of particular attention and are considered in rather more detail below.

Hypertension

The effects of maternal hypertension and the pathology of pre-eclampsia have been the subject of considerable research and remain a subject of debate. The debate is obscured by differences in systems of classification.

Nevertheless, MacGillivray (1967) has shown that women with a degree of hypertension towards the end of pregnancy have heavier babies than those who remain normotensive. Thomson *et al.* (1967) have also shown that a degree of oedema was a positive indication for the birthweight of the baby. The physiological response to pregnancy of increased plasma volume, oedema and mild hypertension seems to be non-pathological although, in many systems of classification, this might be referred to as mild pre-eclampsia.

Severe pre-eclampsia, characterised by substantial proteinuria, however, results in marked growth retardation and increased incidence of perinatal mortality (Baird *et al.*, 1957; Butler and Alberman, 1969; Page and Christianson, 1976). Women with mild essential hypertension who become pregnant have babies of similar weight to the babies of normotensive women but, if the hypertension is severe, birthweight tends to be reduced (Dunlop, 1966).

The joint effects of pre-eclampsia and smoking are the subject of a particular study later in this monograph (chapter 11).

Diabetes

The increased birthweight of babies born to diabetic mothers has been widely documented, one of the earlier reports being that of Pederson (1954). It was later noted (Bolton, 1959) that some women who were not overtly diabetic but who gave birth to excessively large babies developed diabetes in later life, and the term 'gestational diabetes' was coined (O'Sullivan *et al.*, 1966) to refer to women who developed temporary abnormal glucose tolerance during pregnancy. O'Sullivan *et al.* (1973) have confirmed that the babies of gestational diabetics are at risk similarly to the babies of overt diabetics. It appears likely that the excess weight of babies born to diabetic mothers is associated with an increase in the fat stores of such babies (Osler and Pedersen, 1960) and the use of birthweight to assess fetal development for such babies is thus open to doubt.

Maternal smoking habits

The effects of smoking in pregnancy have been extensively reviewed in a recent report of the United States Public Health Service (1979). In common with numerous previous reports (45 of which are reviewed by the Public Health Service report), the adverse effects of maternal cigarette consumption on fetal growth are noted. The average reduction in the weight of babies born to mothers who smoke is about 200 g.

The stage of pregnancy at which smoking is most harmful remains a matter of some debate, but Pirani (1978) argues that it is certainly harmful during the second trimester of pregnancy and probably earlier. Miller and Hassanein (1976) have shown that the effect of smoking is an overall reduction in the baby's size rather than merely an effect on the stores of subcutaneous fat.

Although women who smoke tend to have smaller babies than those who do not, Yerushalmy (1971, 1972, 1974) has argued, in a widely criticised set of studies, that other characteristics of smokers play their part in the observed reduction in birthweight. Suggestions that the effects of maternal smoking overlap with those of social class have appeared in the literature (e.g. Andrews and McGary, 1972).

Nicotine, carbon monoxide, cyanide and thiocyanate may all contribute to the direct effect of smoking on birthweight, and the hypotensive effects of the latter may explain the lower incidence of pre-eclampsia in smokers (Duffus and MacGillivray, 1968). Epidemiological evidence from Aberdeen is reported in a later section of this book (chapters 10 and 11).

Geographic factors

Differences in birthweight between and within particular populations may be explained by factors associated with the location. In particular, it has been suggested that climate may account for some seasonal differences in birthweight. After controlling for other factors, Roberts (1976) has shown that babies born in the hottest season in Hong Kong were about 120 g lighter than those born in the colder months and a similar finding is reported by Selvin and Janerich in New York (1971).

Altitude, too, is a factor affecting birthweight. Sobrevilla *et al.* (1968) report a dramatic reduction with extreme altitude, although the numbers in their survey are very small. McCullough *et al.* (1977) found an association between birthweight and altitude in Colorado, women from the highest locations bearing children on average 200 g lighter than women from Denver. Denver itself is at an altitude of some 1600 m and this fact alone might cast doubt on the applicability of Lubchenco *et al.*'s (1963) standards of fetal growth in locations nearer sea-level. We have argued the need for appropriate 'local' standards elsewhere (Carr-Hill and Pritchard, 1983) and this is the subject of further comment in chapters 5 and 9.

Socio-economic factors

A variety of studies (Thomson *et al.*, 1968 [Aberdeen]); Sibert *et al.*, 1978 [India]; Naeye *et al.*, 1971 [USA]) have documented the tendency for dis-advantaged groups in society to have smaller babies than more advantaged groups. Differences in living standards within a given society may affect birthweight through a number of the factors already noted above and evidence of the relationships between some of these factors, socio-economic status and birthweight is discussed later in this monograph (chapter 11).

Other factors

Many factors other than those discussed above have been reported as affecting birthweight. A wide variety of drugs have been implicated in reductions of birthweight (Adamson and Joelsson, 1977) and the effects of abuse of heroin (Blinick *et al.*, 1976) or alcohol (Ouellette *et al.*, 1977) have been widely reported, although Tennes and Blackard (1980) found no effect of alcohol consumption on birthweight once other confounding factors were controlled. Radiation in the huge doses after the atomic explosions in Japan had, amongst its other devastating effects, the effect of reducing the weight of babies born to women with radiation sickness (Yamazaki *et al.*, 1954).

CONCLUSION

Any review of the literature on factors associated with birthweight is bound to be more or less idiosyncratic; the literature is huge and ever increasing. Not only are there factors which have not been mentioned, but also many of the factors reviewed are themselves complexly related in any pregnancy. Moreover, we have not discussed here the important effects of the clinical management of pregnancy. Not only may such management intervene to mitigate the adverse effects of some of the factors noted above but, as noted in the discussion of induction in chapter 2, it may also directly affect birthweight distributions.

The intention of this chapter, then, has been to outline the main variables affecting birthweight and at least to refer to the literature in which they have been discussed. As such, it provides a background for the theoretical and empirical work which follows.

Particular issues which are the subject of later discussion have been indicated, and certain of the controversies, which have special relevance to the development of birthweight standards, have been noted. It is, however, important to stress that the evidence presented in section 2 of the book is not intended to resolve the issues addressed. The studies are based on a particular population over a particular time-span. Not only does geographical location influence the patterns observed but there has also been a marked secular trend in birthweight-for-gestation over the last twenty years (see chapter 2). While the findings presented may throw some light on certain aspects of the problems, the purpose of this book is not to provide a universally applicable predictive model of birthweight but rather to argue for (and illustrate) a particular approach to the development of appropriate *local* birthweight standards.

4

Birthweight surveys

INTRODUCTION

The longstanding interest in establishing the 'normal range' of birthweight has resulted in a considerable number of surveys of birthweight. Meredith's (1970) review of some 230 surveys represents only a fraction of those that were available at the time, and publication of the results of surveys has continued apace. Surveys differ in size, quality of data collection, sampling methods and intentions. The purpose of this review is to consider survey practice in three respects: firstly to examine what variables have been regularly used in the analysis of birthweight surveys; secondly the choice of a population; and thirdly the criteria for inclusion of births in surveys. Since this monograph is principally concerned with methods of estimating and understanding the normal range of birthweights and their implications, surveys which have been exclusively concerned with births beyond the normal range have not been considered.

FACTORS CONSIDERED IN THE ANALYSIS OF BIRTHWEIGHT SURVEYS

As noted in the previous chapter, there are many factors which influence birthweight. Among surveys of birthweight, the extent to which these factors are considered varies considerably, reflecting differences in the reasons for which the surveys were conducted.

Gestation

The majority of birthweight surveys analyse birthweight in terms of gestation. Some surveys (e.g. Naeye and Dixon, 1978) have focussed on birthweight for gestation exclusively.

Sex of infant

Most surveys, too, analyse their results in terms of the sex of the infant. Gesta-

38

tion and sex were the two factors considered by Lubchenco *et al.* (1963) whose standards are widely used in clinical practice.

Parity

Parity is also commonly taken into account in the assessment of the normal range of birthweight so that the analysis of birthweight data by gestation, sex and parity groups as presented by Thomson *et al.* (1968) represents a standard pattern for many surveys.

Maternal age

The persistent controversy surrounding the effects of maternal age has ensured its frequent inclusion among the factors considered in birthweight surveys from Donald's (1938) early survey onwards.

Maternal size

The factors considered so far are factors which may be routinely collected in birth registration or hospital records. For retrospective studies, the consideration of the parameters of maternal size depends to some extent on the availability of data. Most commonly, it is maternal height which is considered (Barron and Vessey, 1966; McKeown and Record, 1954), although the effects of both height and weight have been analysed in many studies (e.g. Love and Kinch, 1965; Rush *et al.*, 1972). O'Sullivan *et al.* (1973) considered weight alone.

Ethnic origin

Several studies have been concerned to establish the normal range of birthweight for different ethnic groups, notably Brenner *et al.* (1976) and Cheng *et al.* (1972).

Maternal disease

The diseases most commonly considered in birthweight surveys are pre-eclamptic toxaemia (e.g. Butler and Alberman, 1969) and diabetes (e.g. North *et al.*, 1977).

Maternal social status

The mother's socio-economic status, as represented by the Registrar General's Social Class classification, has been used in the analysis of birthweight surveys in Britain (e.g. Butler and Alberman, 1969; Thomson *et al.*, 1968) and Ireland (Dowding, 1981). Dougherty and Jones (1982) used maternal occupation and accommodation variables in their assessment of the effects of socio-economic status.

Summary

In general, then, many of the factors believed to affect birthweight (see previous chapters) have found their place in the analysis of surveys of birthweight. The position to be adopted in the analyses later in this book is argued in detail with respect to the derivation of an account of the normal range of birthweight in recent years in Aberdeen in chapter 5. However, the important point to note here is the relative consistency of the use of gestation, sex and parity and the relative inconsistency with respect to other factors.

CHOOSING A POPULATION

Birthweight surveys, including those which have resulted in standards for the range of normal birthweight are in widespread use and are based on particular samples from particular populations. The definition of the population has important substantive and statistical implications (as was demonstrated in chapter 2). There are a variety of ways of choosing a population: in practice, in most birthweight surveys, two methods have tended to predominate.

Geographical selection

Inevitably, surveys of birthweight have drawn their samples from within one geographically defined area. Thus, for example, Fraccaro's (1958) sample was from Czechoslovakia and the British Perinatal Mortality Surveys (e.g. Butler and Alberman, 1969) were national. More commonly, a particular location with a country is selected, as in the case of Selvin and Janerich's (1971) New York survey or Kloosterman's (1970) study of births in Amsterdam and Thomson *et al.*'s (1968) study of Aberdeen City. Drawing a sample from a geographical area has the advantage of controlling for a variety of possibly confounding factors including, for example, altitude and climate which were noted in the previous chapter. Occasionally, as with Thomson *et al.* (1968), the geographical criterion has been used to provide a notional total population as a basis from which to draw the sample. In some places, where virtually all deliveries occur in one hospital, such selection is obviously equivalent to geographic selection in providing a 'complete' population as a basis for samples. More usually, however, the situation is more complicated. In fact, it would be rare for the catchment of one hospital among several to constitute a sample representative of any meaningful geographical population.

Selection by place of confinement

Commonly, too, surveys of birthweight are based on births occurring in a particular hospital (e.g. Gruenwald, 1966; Rush *et al.*, 1972). For example, the Aberdeen Maternity Hospital provides obstetric services for women resident in

Aberdeen City and district and additionally for women living outside the immediate catchment area whose pregnancy or delivery requires particular care. In many large cities, however, a particular hospital serves only one fairly well-defined location within the city which may be biased in ethnic or socio-economic composition relative to the city as a whole. Moreover, in some cultures, as Mosely and Knox (1960) noted in the case of Western Nigeria, only a minority of births occur in hospital.

There are, however, important advantages of selecting one place of confinement. In the first place, gynaecological and obstetric practices are more likely to be consistent. For example, the influence of differences in induction practice over time has been noted in chapter 2. Particular patterns of antenatal care probably have particular effects. Secondly, uniformity of measurement and coding practice are more probable and this represents a special advantage of clarity in analysis.

SAMPLING CRITERIA FOR INCLUSION IN BIRTHWEIGHT SURVEYS

The utility of standards derived from a particular survey sample, for populations other than those from which the sample was drawn, ultimately depends on the extent to which the sample can be taken as representative of other populations. This issue is the subject of special consideration, both with respect to the general form and particular estimates of the effects of factors incorporated in standards, in chapters 7, 8 and 12. Nevertheless, given the inevitable sensitivity of standards to their origins, it is, perhaps, surprising that criteria for population selection show such diversity, and the purpose of the following review is to attempt to bring out some of the salient issues.

Certainty of gestation

The majority of recent surveys have been concerned to analyse birthweight for gestation and, as such, it has appeared desirable to include only births where gestation is known with some quantifiable degree of accuracy. Thus, for example, Thomson *et al.* (1968) excluded births where gestation was 'not known', but included births where a 'best estimate' of gestational age was possible. The exclusion of unsure gestations removes an avoidable source of error even though such a procedure may introduce a bias where uncertainty of gestation is associated with factors which may influence birthweight, for example, the mother's socio-economic status.

Work by our obstetric colleagues in Aberdeen (vide Hall *et al.*, 1984) has shown that the estimate of gestation is of doubtful accuracy in a far larger proportion of births than is usually acknowledged. They have also demonstrated the importance of distinguishing between an accurate estimate of gestation (supra) and a clinical assessment of the reliability of that estimate. The significance of these arguments in studies of birthweight-for-gestation is discussed in chapter 5. Ideally, of course, the assessment of the reliability of the estimate of gestational age used as a criterion for the inclusion or exclusion of births from a sample in a survey of birthweights ought not to depend at all on parameters of the baby's size (see chapters 5 and 6).

Fetal malformations

Some congenital disorders, for example anencephaly, have a direct effect on birthweight, and the exclusion of cases of gross fetal abnormality is common practice in birthweight surveys (e.g. Thomson *et al.*, 1968), although some samples (e.g. Kloosterman, 1970) include such births. Some surveys exclude all births where there was a lethal condition present at birth (e.g. Love and Kinch, 1965) and Naeye and Dixon (1978) excluded all cases where the infant did not survive its first year.

Stillbirths

Some surveys (e.g. Lubchenco *et al.*, 1963; Battaglia *et al.*, 1966) exclude all stillbirths. Others include only unmacerated stillbirths (e.g. Thomson *et al.*, 1968) or stillbirths where death occurred less than three days prior to birth (e.g. Kloosterman, 1970) or stillbirths where death occurred in the course of labour (Brenner *et al.*, 1976). Yet other surveys (e.g. Selvin and Janerich, 1971) include all births whether live or still.

Maternal disease

While most surveys include both normal and pathological pregnancies in their sample some exclude cases of maternal disease. Some exclusions have been maternal diabetes and pre-eclampsia (e.g. Hendricks, 1964), rhesus incompatibility (e.g. Brenner *et al.*, 1976), syphilis (Kassius *et al.*, 1958) and, most sweeping of all, 'any medical, surgical or obstetrical complication of pregnancy' (Love and Kinch, 1965).

Multiple pregnancy

By far the majority of surveys are for singleton pregnancies, a large exception being Fraccaro's (1958) survey.

Statistical criteria

One reason for excluding cases is that there are very few cases in a particular cell. Thus, for example, births before 28 weeks gestation (e.g. Selvin and Janerich, 1971) or after 42 weeks gestation (e.g. Lubchenco *et al.*, 1963) are commonly excluded because of the small numbers born at those weeks. The statistical method employed may involve the exclusion of births for which some of the data are missing, for example, the analysis of variance employed by Butler and Alberman (1969) involved (at least) the deletion of cases for those variables used in the analysis. Dougherty and Jones (1982) exclude 'extreme cases' on the grounds that their inclusion may violate the homoscedasicity assumption required by regression analyses.

Others

Some surveys (e.g. Lubchenco *et al.*, 1963; Barron and Vessey, 1966) exclude some births on the grounds of ethnic origin. Other surveys exclude some cases on (apparently) idiosyncratic grounds, for example, Thomson *et al.*'s (1968) exclusion of illegitimate births.

Summary

Overall, then, the criteria by which cases are included or excluded in a birth-weight survey shows considerable variation. Where the intention of the survey is to provide estimates of the 'normal' range of birthweight, it appears appropriate to exclude cases of gross abnormality involving the loss of organs, such as anencephaly, or the maceration of a stillborn fetus since such cases clearly do not represent 'normality'. Whether 'abnormal' might be extended to include the babies of, for example, diabetic mothers is less certain. Indeed, the whole question of 'normality' is central to the argument presented in the next chapter. However, what is clear is that it is incumbent upon reports of surveys to be very specific about the selection criteria employed and to consider the implications of exclusions. As the number and variety of cases excluded increases so does the potential for bias and it would be helpful if surveys were to attempt an empirical assessment of the bias introduced as far as possible. The criteria used in the survey reported later in this book are discussed and evaluated in chapter 6.

5
The theory, the model, an analytic strategy

INTRODUCTION

The preceding two chapters have demonstrated a wide measure of agreement as to the direction of the effects of the various factors influencing birthweight. On the other hand, the review of birthweight surveys (like this one) shows no general agreement as to the relative importance or even priority among or between groups of factors, whose effects upon birthweight often overlap. For example, a comparison of two recent sets of data from Scotland – Forbes and Smalls (1983) based on Glasgow births, and Carr-Hill and Pritchard (1983), based on the Aberdeen data used in this monograph – reveal only broad similarities in mean birthweight for gestation and the relative magnitude and significance of effects. The purpose of this chapter is, therefore, to explore whether or not it is (theoretically) possible to develop a general model of the process determining birthweight and to examine the implications for both understanding and analysis.

Why the enthusiasm for a model? There are several reasons, on different levels. On one level, a model which both reflects theory and represents observations is intellectually satisfying. Unfortunately, the review of the literature makes this seem unlikely: there is no general theory of fetal growth and most studies record a large unexplained variance on birthweight. On another level, a working model is a useful tool for resolving problems: in this case, for example, it might help us to understand why the birthweight distribution has a consistently high standard deviation at all gestational ages. On yet another, more pragmatic and technical level, a plausible model will inform the choice of analytic strategy and of statistical techniques so as to obtain reliable and repeatable statistical estimates of the parameters of that model. In the absence of a complete model which would dictate the appropriate analytic strategy, the choice of approach to analysis is much more complicated. This chapter, therefore, first explores the possibility of developing a model before discussing the approach to analysis.

A MODEL FOR THE DETERMINATION OF BIRTHWEIGHT

In principle, the problem is deceptively simple: the weight of a newborn baby is an observation at one point of a process of fetal growth. Where there are enough observations at different gestational ages, so as to control statistically for the effects of disturbing random factors, then it should be possible to estimate the parameters of the fetal growth process. So all that is required according to this story is to separate the factors into two groups: those which are integral to the fetal growth process, and those which disturb that process. In the former category, there are factors such as sex and parity which characterise and influence every fetal growth process; in the latter category there are diseases of pregnancy such as pre-eclampsia and maternal diabetes which clearly are perturbations specific to only some pregnancies. It is less clear what should be the status of parameters of maternal conformation such as height and weight.

That kind of problem is, however, in principle, theoretically resolvable and a 'standard' birthweight would be the outcome of entering the actual values for the first category of factors specific to this pregnancy into the formula for fetal growth and the observed birthweight could then be referred to that 'standard'. Research would concentrate on the effect of diseases of pregnancy upon birthweight and on the effect of socio-demographic factors such as social class and civil status upon the distribution of maternal characteristics and the incidence of these diseases of maternal pregnancy. This story is illustrated in figure 5.1.

The story is, unfortunately, incomplete: the weight of a newborn baby depends not only on the rate of fetal growth but also upon the length of gestation; and the determinants of the onset of labour are less well known. Thus, although 'birthweight is usually thought of as a function of the length of gestation, it is equally plausible that the length of gestation is determined by the weight of the fetus or by some factor related to weight, such as organ maturation' (Wilcox, 1981). Wilcox (1981) goes on to argue that the classical hypothesis of a fetal growth curve which is affected by a variety of maternal characteristics (e.g. ethnic origin, smoking habits) in the last trimester of pregnancy does not account for the data and that 'anomalous' birthweight distributions are better understood in terms of shifts in the *bivariate* distribution of birthweight and gestational age.

Most importantly, this latter story implies that a curve of birthweight by gestation does not literally describe the fetal growth process, in that a pre-term birth may not be typical of the average unborn fetus at this age. *In extremis*, every birth is the result of a unique fetal growth process. The purpose of developing a model is to detect and describe the similarities across births. The implications of this for the model proposed in figure 5.1 mean that the model to be estimated takes the form of figure 5.2, in which fetal growth is conceptualised as growth rate per week. The *pattern* of growth, taken in conjunction with the gestational age at which spontaneous labour commences, determines, rather than is measured by, birthweight.

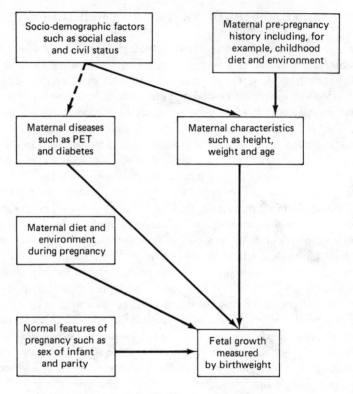

Figure 5.1   Modelling the fetal growth process

The model is clearly more complex: the question is whether or not it is possible to estimate the parameters of this process (or the path coefficients of this model). Theoretically, yes: the system is recursive with:

(1)   bwt = f_1 (gest, fgr)
(2)   gest = f_2 (fgr, mat char, mat dis)
(3)   fgr = f_3 (norm feat, mat char, mat dis, mat dep)
(4) mat char = f_4 (diet, environment)

where bwt = birthweight, fgr = fetal growth rate, gest = gestational age, mat = maternal characteristics, mat dis = maternal disease, mat dep = maternal diet and environment during pregnancy, norm feat = normal features of pregnancy.

Theoretically possible, but statistically difficult as the fetal growth rate is usually unobserved. With the improvements of ultrasound scanning, of course, possibilities open up a direct and non-invasive monitoring of fetal growth. As far as the authors are aware, the frequent and regular monitoring entailed has not been carried out for a large enough sample (but see Dobbing and Sands, 1978; Campbell 1976).

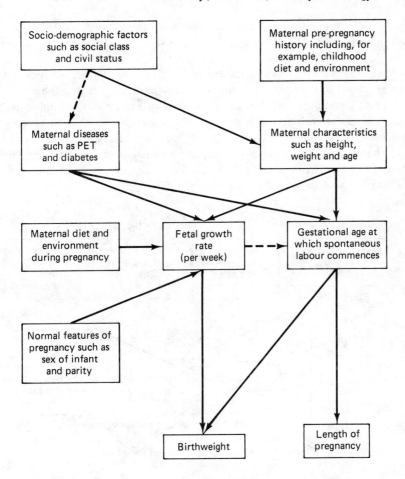

Figure 5.2   Modelling birthweight

At present, moreover, there is an added complication: it is not obvious that gestational age can be measured without error. There are obvious reasons for this, ranging from uncertainties about dates on the part of the mother (Hall *et al.*, 1984) to the possibility of confusing vaginal bleeding in early pregnancy with the last menstrual period (see Naeye and Dixon, 1978). A variety of solutions have been proposed in the literature involving the exclusion of those infants who are older than their calculated gestational ages: thus, Lubchenco *et al.* (1963) used a scattergram and review of clinical course, whilst Usher and MacLean (1969) added clinical tests of the neonate's maturity. However, as Naeye and Dixon (1978) rightly point out, any such procedure is very unsatisfactory because relatively arbitrary. They propose the use of a probability plot method, wherein they retain only the lowest birthweight cluster for any given gestational age on the presumption that there has been confusion between vaginal bleeding and menstruation. This procedure has the advantage of reducing the standard deviation at each gestational age considerably.

Superficially, this procedure is attractive, especially as it deals with one of the puzzles about birthweight distribution — their consistently high standard deviation at all gestational ages. But at best, it only takes care of one kind of uncertainty in gestational age. Hall *et al.* (1984) argue instead that all sources of possible error in the estimation of gestation should be systematically explored and that a division between certain, approximate and uncertain gestations discriminates between pregnancy outcomes. Their discussion would imply a *measurement* model for gestation as shown in figure 5.3.

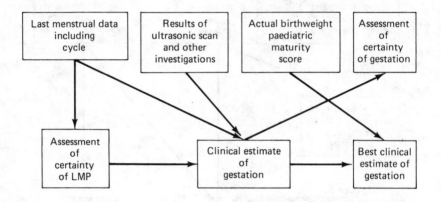

Figure 5.3   Measurement model for gestation

The trouble is that the combination of this measurement model with the substantive model in figure 5.2 leads, in general, to a system of equations which is not identified. Figure 5.3 is equivalent to adding a further equation to the system f_1, f_2, f_3 and f_4 of the form:

(5) gest $= h_1$ (clin est, char of neonate)

and, insofar as neonatal characteristics are dominated by the observed birthweight, the system f_1, f_2, f_3, f_4 and h_i is not identified (for an explanation of this technical term see Hanushek and Jackson, 1977). This can be seen as follows: if we solve f_1, f_2, f_3 and f_4 for fgr which is unobservable, we obtain:

(6) bwt $= f_5$ (gest, norm feat, mat char, mat dis)
(7) gest $= f_6$ (norm feat, mat char, mat dis)
(8) gest $= h_1$ (clin est, bwt)

If (7) and (8) are combined — as they must be for the purposes of estimation — to form

(9) gest = h_2 (clin est, bwt, norm feat, mat char, mat dis)

then equation (6) cannot be distinguished from the more inclusive equation (9). Formally, one of the necessary conditions for identification — that each equation contains at least one variable not in the other equations — is absent. The problem is that birthweight is a function of gestation and observed gestation is a function of birthweight.

In an ideal world, of course, ultrasound measurements would replace other procedures for estimating gestation, equation (5) would be irrelevant and the simpler system of figure 5.3 holds. Unfortunately, the world is not ideal and the use of ultrasound to estimate gestation would depend on standards having already been derived, with exactly the same attendant problems in estimating gestation. The overall implication of this argument is that the *structural parameters** of the process of fetal growth cannot be identified.

The only way out of the dilemma is if the functional form h_1 of equation (5) does not apply. In turn, this is only true if the recorded values for gestation do not depend upon measurements upon the size of the neonate. In the Aberdeen context, this means restricting the sample to those for whom the best clinical estimate of gestational age is assessed as 'certain'. For although the birthweight and paediatric maturity scores are taken into account in the estimate of gestation in *all* cases, in cases which are assessed as 'certain' the birthweight and paediatric maturity scores simply *confirm* other evidence, whilst cases which are assessed as 'approximate' or 'uncertain' indicate a disagreement between different kinds of evidence (including evidence of neonatal characteristics).

Restriction to those with 'certain' gestational ages, therefore, does not, in general, lead to the difficulties of inference discussed above. However, note that if neonatal size were to be used in the assessment of certainty then, once again, some high or low birthweights would be excluded basically because they are high or low and this would lead to an underestimation of variability.

The restriction to the 'certain' group of cases in the Aberdeen context therefore allows us to replace the functional form h_1 in equation (5) with

(10) gest = clin est

---

* Structural parameters is a technical term referring to the relatively unmixed, invariant autonomous features of the system which generate the observed variables of the sort which are estimated in structural equation models (see Duncan, 1975).

Working backwards, this means that the system (6), (7) and (8) can be replaced by:

(11)   bwt $= f^1_5$ (gest, norm feat, mat char, mat dis)

(12)   gest $= f^1_6$ (norm feat, mat char, mat dis)

We have apparently arrived at a recursive system, the structural parameter of which could be estimated. However, equation (12) looks remarkably like equation (3) — the equation for the fetal growth rate. For, whilst the precise functional form is, in principle, different, because of the substitutions, etc., the actual estimation involves exactly the same variables. Because fetal growth rate can, in practice, only be observed as achieved birthweight, this effectively means that, for the purposes of estimating the parameters of this system, gestation has to be treated as a function of birthweight. In practice, therefore, whilst not in theory, the system remains unidentified.

We are, therefore, forced to estimate the equations separately. In this monograph the focus, of course, is on the equation for birthweight. It is important to emphasise that, even when estimating this equation separately, the simultaneity which arises from the problem of measuring gestation must still be circumvented by the restriction to certain gestations.

Note that there are apparently similar difficulties with the *measurement* of maternal weight independently of birthweight. For, in the majority of studies — including this one (see chapter 6) — the mother is weighed during pregnancy and so, inevitably, fetal growth will have contributed to her observed weight. However, the problem is not as severe as with gestation: first, it is, in principle, avoidable by weighing a representative population of potential mothers; secondly, even though that is probably impracticable, the extent of the problem can be precisely quantified — how much weight do mothers actually gain during pregnancy? The introduction of a measurement model for maternal weight therefore seems unnecessarily complex: instead, precautions are taken to record data on maternal weight at a standard gestational age and as early as possible in pregnancy (see chapter 6).

Each of the other observed variables, also in principle, are subject to measurement error. However, the problems are by no means as severe as those considered above.

The problems in developing a model that have arisen in this section have, therefore, been circumvented, but the status of the resulting model is rather different from the original grand design in which the structural parameters of a fetal growth process were being identified. In the first place, the argument that there was not one fetal growth process but a whole family of processes characterised by the joint distribution of birthweight and gestation, means that the observed 'birthweight for gestation' curve is a specific mix from that family of processes, and the specific mix has to be empirically determined in each population. In the second place, the measurement problem means that the estimation of reliable and stable parameters depends upon the choice of a sample defined by hospital-specific criteria for assessing the certainty of gestation. Given these two caveats, the standards derived by any statistical processes can only be appropriate to particular populations at particular times (see also Forbes and Smalls, 1983, and chapter 2).

TYPES OF FACTORS AFFECTING BIRTHWEIGHT

The previous chapter has shown how there is little consensus as to which of the factors associated with birthweight ought to be taken into account in deriving standards. At the beginning of the previous section (p. 45) a crude division, for the purposes of developing the argument about the model, was adopted. On the one hand, there were 'integral' factors representing the likeness between unique fetal processes and, on the other hand, there were specific and particular 'disturbances' of that process. The purpose of this section is to clarify and document that dichotomy.

It is easier to understand the distinction in terms of the purposes of developing standards. The introductory chapter showed how the development of standards for clinical or for research purposes meant that the status of the standards would be different. In the case of clinical standards, the concept of normality refers to the population on the basis of which the standards were derived; in the case of research standards the concept of normality depends on the factors of interest to the researcher.

Whilst there clearly are differences in the perception of normality, we would argue that in both cases there is the basic distinction between two kinds of factors influencing birthweight — 'normal' and 'non-normal'. We shall define 'normal' factors as those factors which are a feature of every pregnancy and where the associated decrement or increment in *fetal growth rate* does not of itself influence the prognosis for the baby or future pregnancies of the mother. Typically, variations in the fetal growth rate arising from genetic differences in the heritability of size as between, say, male and female babies or racial groups would fall into this category. We define 'non-normal' factors as those which may or may not occur and where there is *prima facie* evidence to suppose that the associated decrement or increment in the fetal growth rate in itself influences the prognosis for the baby or future pregnancies of the mother. Typically, one would include pre-eclampsia and smoking habits in this category. In general, both clinical and research standards will incorporate 'normal factors' and will not standardise for 'non-normal' factors. Unfortunately, this dichotomous division cannot be maintained as there are ambiguities in the classification of some influencing factors and these we shall call intermediate factors.

'Intermediate' factors are those present in every pregnancy but where the effects on growth rate may themselves influence prognosis or where the effects are confounded with the effects of 'non-normal' factors. Important differences in the development of birthweight standards for clinical or for research purposes are more likely to arise in respect of these 'intermediate' factors. Their inclusions in either type of standards is discussed on a case by case basis below. Their status relative to each other is considered in chapter 9.

'Normal' factors

Gestation

Clearly, the effects of being born pre-term may influence the prognosis for the baby. However, gestation-specific changes in *growth rate* do not, of themselves, influence the prognosis of any particular weight or gestation and are hence considered 'normal'.

Sex

The sex of the baby is considered a 'normal' factor since, for example, it is not suggested that the lightness of female relative to male babies represents a form of growth retardation. It is noteworthy that only these two factors are routinely used for the assessment of fetal growth in Sweden. One would argue that gestation and sex specific standards represent a minimum for clinically useful standards.

'Intermediate' factors

Parity

Parity is, of course, a feature of every pregnancy and it is well-established that first born are lighter than later born at all gestational ages. However, it could just be argued that the smaller fetal growth rate associated with primaparity represents a departure from the 'normal' pattern of fetal growth which has similar features and prognosis for the baby, to other forms of growth retardation (see, for example, chapter 2). Further, grand multiparity in many populations, including Aberdeen, is closely related to socio-economic status which may confound the observed effects.

For clinical purposes, standards developed on the basis of gestational age, sex of infant, and maternal parity are conventional; for research purposes, insofar as the effects of parity are not the object of research, such standards would usually be appropriate. In this sense, therefore, parity is the most 'normal' of the intermediate factors.

Maternal size

Maternal size may be considered as a normal factor insofar as it represents a genetically determined feature of the mother and may be reflected in the genetically determined growth of her baby. But the evidence of inter-generational studies is that the relation between the pregnancy outcomes of mother and daughter is weak (see Robson, 1955; and the discussion in chapter 12). More-over, the stature and weight of the mother is influenced by, for example, her diet during childhood, adolescence and adulthood, or by disease which may, in turn, influence the fetal growth of her baby. Indeed, as Morton (1955) and a variety of animal studies (e.g. Joubert and Hammond, 1954) have suggested, maternal size may represent a purely or principally 'environmental' constraint on fetal growth.

In general, maternal height which is relatively stable over a woman's repro-ductive career, may be a better reflection of the mother's genetic characteristics than maternal weight, which is subject to short-term variation dependent, for example, on eating habits. Also, if, as is usual, maternal weight is measured during pregnancy, the observed weight will include some proportion due to the effects of pregnancy itself. As was explained in the previous section, this may seriously confound the interpretation of any observed covariation between maternal weight or maternal weight-for-height and birthweight.

In common with Thomson *et al.* (1968) the clinical standards developed in chapter 9 present corrections for maternal height and for maternal weight-for-height. The extent to which these corrections *ought* to influence clinical judgement, however, remains an open question (see Discussion in chapters 9 and 12). For the purposes of research, the incorporation of corrections for maternal height and for maternal weight-for-height depends obviously on their relevance and priority in respect of the specific research questions being addressed, but also on the form which the corrections take.

Ethnic origin

Ethnic origin is considered a 'normal' factor in that it represents a genetic influence on fetal growth. However, differences in, for example, life-style and nutrition between different ethnic groups represent major confounding features. The complex effects of different ethnic mixes in the different parents are, more-over, difficult to quantify. In Aberdeen, where the population is of relatively homogeneous ethnic origins, it is not possible to address the issue of ethnic origin in either clinical or research standards.

Where data are available, the development of standards specific to a particu-lar racial group for clinical purposes may be technically feasible; whether or not it is appropriate will depend upon many other factors. Similarly, whilst it may be helpful for researchers to be aware of the distribution of different racial groups in the population since the variation in birthweight associated with differences in ethnic origin may confound other analyses (quite apart from any research interest in the effects of ethnic origin itself), there might be difficulties in collecting the data.

Maternal age

While maternal age is a factor common to all pregnancies, it may be that, for example, the relative lightness of babies born to younger mothers represents a departure from 'normal' fetal growth. The age at which mothers start their child-bearing careers is closely related to socio-economic status (for Aberdeen data see Pritchard and Thompson, 1982) and because of the close association between maternal age and parity, it is difficult to assess the independent effects of maternal age. In deriving birthweight standards for clinical or research use, it is suggested that the effects of maternal age should be examined closely in the way illustrated in chapters 7 and 8.

'Non-normal' factors

Other factors discussed in chapter 3 are considered 'non-normal'. Clearly, maternal diseases occurring during pregnancy such as pre-eclampsia and gesta-tional diabetes are 'non-normal'. They only occur to a relatively small proportion of mothers and they are known to influence the fetal growth rate certainly in late pregnancy. The status of more general maternal characteristics (such as socio-economic status) or habits (such as smoking) is much less clear. Every mother has a socio-economic status and, at least in this population, many mothers-to-be smoke or have smoked during pregnancy. Whilst, therefore, factors such as being underprivileged and/or smoking during pregnancy may well have deleterious effects on fetal growth, which is why they have been classified as 'non-normal' factors — they are clearly not statistically atypical phenomena. The problem arises because, obviously, the distribution of non-normal factors in a particular population is unique to that population and, therefore, the effects of these factors on the distribution of birthweight are peculiar to the particular population, by virtue of their unique distribution (see chapter 2).

For research purposes, this is not critical and in some circumstances may even be helpful. The effects of particular 'non-normal' factors may be controlled for or examined in the specific populations in their own right, depending on the research questions addressed.

In a clinical context, however, 'non-normal' factors like these present some-thing of a dilemma. For example, it might be that the babies of smokers are on average 150 g lighter than the babies of non-smokers. If half the population smoke, the babies of non-smokers will, on average, be 75 g heavier than the standard and the babies of smokers, on average, 75 g lighter. This would mean that the babies of non-smokers would have to be that much lighter than the normal range for non-smokers to be considered light-for-dates while the delete-rious effects of smoking would be under-estimated by reference to the standard.

Induction practice, too, has particular effects on the distribution of birth-weight in a particular population. Although induction does not affect the fetal growth rate, and is therefore anomalous within the classification developed here, it has particular effects at particular points in the distribution of birthweight for gestation. As discussed in chapter 2, induction is a response to a clinical assess-ment of the progress of the pregnancy and hence, at least in major part, a response to an assessment of the development of the fetus. This is especially apparent in the relative lightness of pre-term induced babies compared to those born after a spontaneous onset of labour at the same gestation. In the same way as commented upon in the case of smoking, this would mean that non-induced babies would have to be lighter than the normal range for spontaneous births to be considered light-for-dates and the appropriateness of induction under-estimated by reference to the standard.

The alternative, however, would be to derive clinical standards for non-induced babies born to non-smoking, disease-free, higher social status, well-nourished women living at sea level in temperate climates; but 'standards' could then only reflect the fetal growth process among these particular women. While such standards might represent a step in the derivation of some notional universal model for fetal growth, the argument in the previous section of this chapter would suggest that this would be unlikely: it would indeed be fortuitous if this particular subgroup of the population (non-smoking, disease-free, etc. . .) were also homogeneous in respect of the pattern of fetal growth they followed.

Note that none of this constitutes an argument against standardisation *per se*. The point is that there is a distinction between developing a set of standards (for a particular population at a particular time) and standardising or controlling for extraneous factors. Clearly, we must *standardise* for gestation, sex, parity, etc., when analysing birth outcomes. The issue here is which partic-ular set of factors *in any given context* should be incorporated (via standardisa-tion) into a proposed set of standards.

Indeed, all population based empirical standards like those derived in chapters 7 and 8, represent the normal range of birthweight in a particular population with a particular distribution of non-normal factors. Their clinical utility lies in their capacity to indicate departures from that normal range (see also chapters 9 and 12).

GENERAL APPROACH TO ANALYSIS

The title of this section is rather grandiose. The intention is simply to set out the kinds of procedures that should be followed in deriving population based em-pirical standards. For, in the absence of a complete, identified model including a functional form of fetal growth — for which linear structural modelling tech-niques have been developed (see Joreskog and Sorbom 1979) — the approach has to be much more pragmatic.

Decisions about the base population and independent variables incorporated in the analysis

Since standards are to be derived empirically, some care is needed in thinking about the nature of the population and the variables to be used in the analysis.

As noted, both population and variables are constrained by the available data and, beyond that, particular research questions may further define the appropriate population upon which standards should be based in the context of a particular piece of work. This section addresses more general issues than those which would be considered in a particular research design.

A preliminary analysis of any data set ought to consist in the sort of general familiarisation with the distributions of the variables, such as the descriptive statistics for the Aberdeen material presented in chapter 6 and its Data Appendix. Beyond that, it is helpful:

(1) Firstly, to take note of whether the population is relatively homogeneous in terms of the variables which are *not* to be included in the analysis in order to understand the eventual biases which might arise. An example is 'certainty of gestation', commented upon above and in chapter 6.

(2) Secondly, if any 'peculiar' characteristics of the population are noted, an explanation of differences ought to be sought before conducting complex analyses. An example of this might be the failure to find the 'known' positive association between birthweight and parity in a particular population.

(3) Thirdly, to make some preliminary decisions about what variables to incorporate in the analysis and the form they ought to take.

One insightful and useful way of examining the data with these objectives in mind will be illustrated. The method used is relatively simple and involves the examination of the correlation coefficients between birthweight and those variables which may influence birthweight.

Analytic strategy

Given a large enough population and considerable computational power, it would be possible to standardise birthweight in every cell defined by the cross classification of 'normal' and 'intermediate' factors (see above). However, such a solution is not practical for most populations given the number and form of the independent variables being considered. The aim of the analysis reported in chapters 7 and 8 is thus to reduce the complexity by deriving a statistical model which represents a close approximation to such a standardisation.

Nevertheless, because the aim is essentially descriptive and the approach empirical, a careful balance needs to be struck between the elegance and parsimony of the statistical model and the complexity of the distributions described. The analysis needs to proceed step by step, referring back at each stage to the raw data and 'known' relationships. The process of building an empirical model is an iterative one, moving back and forth between the real world and data, paying due attention to the statistical effects of any simplification.

The details of the analytic procedure are argued for in chapters 7 and 8, but the general stages of analysis are as follows.

Dispensing with independent variables

The first step is to see how far it might be possible to simplify the description by reducing the number of independent variables. Some such reductions are prescribed by the nature of the population under consideration. In Aberdeen, for example, the population is relatively ethnically homogeneous, and an analysis of the effects of ethnic origin is not possible. Of the other intermediate factors, the strength and stability of the association between birthweight and parity, maternal height and weight-for-height suggests that their exclusion would be inappropriate. The effects of maternal age, however, are the subject of particular examination (see chapter 8).

Reducing the range of a variable

A variable, as originally recorded:

    may have been measured more precisely than is warranted by the procedure for collecting data; or
    it may have a very skewed distribution; or
    there may be no difference in effect between several of the levels.

In this study, a classic example of the first is smoking habits, where the raw data is a self-reported consumption rate (but see chapters 10 and 11). A good example of both the second and third is parity which, as originally recorded in the Aberdeen data, may take values from 0 to 10 — with very few women at the higher parities and where the effects of increasing parity are unknown. The analysis explores whether it is possible to treat some of the levels as similar (see chapter 8).

A functional form for gestation

The covariation of birthweight and gestation is one of the central theoretical problems advanced in this monograph. Apart from its theoretical interest, however, it would be very convenient for the construction of birthweight standards if the bivariate relation between, at least the means, could be summarised in a functional form. This, then, should be and is the focus of the first stage of the 'real' analysis (see chapter 7).

Standardising for gestation, sex and parity

Given that the preceding step was unsuccessful, standardised birthweight scores should be derived by referring each birthweight to the mean and standard deviation of its corresponding cell. Standards derived statistically in this way for cells defined by gestation, sex and parity are analysed to ensure that they do 'control' for the effects of gestation, sex and parity (see the beginning of chapter 8).

The effects of other intermediate factors

The residual variation in these standardised birthweight scores are then analysed in terms of the remaining 'intermediate' factors. It is to be expected that the parameters of maternal conformation such as maternal height and weight-for-height would have most effect upon the residual sum of squares. It would then be appropriate to incorporate corrections for maternal height and weight with the standards (see chapter 8), although it remains necessary to check for the effects of maternal age and, where appropriate, ethnic origin.

SECTION 3

The derivation of birthweight standards

The three chapters in this section are devoted to illustrating the derivation of empirical birthweight standards using material from Aberdeen. Chapter 6 describes the Aberdeen Sample and chapters 7 and 8 demonstrate the conceptual and technical work entailed in deriving standards.

6
Material and statistical methods

INTRODUCTION

As with all retrospective analyses, the analysis of birthweight in Aberdeen which occupies the remainder of this book is constrained in a variety of ways by the nature of the data and the statistical techniques which are available. This chapter is concerned to describe these constraints. In the first section the 'involuntary' selection criteria of location, recording and epoch are described. The nature of the variables available for consideration in the ensuing analyses and the criteria used in the selection of a final sample of births are discussed in the second section.

The final section documents the statistical methods which are used in the remainder of this monograph.

THE CHOICE OF A POPULATION FOR THIS SURVEY

Location

The sample is based on births occurring in Aberdeen Maternity Hospital and its associated nursing homes (AMH). As already noted, these provide obstetric services for women resident in Aberdeen city and district and additionally for women whose pregnancy or delivery requires particular care who live outside the immediate catchment area. It is, therefore, essentially a 'hospital population' (see chapter 4). We could have restricted the analysis to Aberdeen District only (cf. Thomson *et al.*, 1968) but we have preferred to use a hospital population as a basis because, having assured ourselves that there was little difference between births to women in Aberdeen District and all births in AMH, the advantages of larger numbers for this illustrative exercise outweigh any possible biases introduced.

The area covered is both urban and rural. Aberdeen itself is at sea-level and there are no extremes of altitude in the area. The climate is temperate with relatively low rainfall, although tends to be colder than more southerly locations in Britain. The crucial point is, of course, that the altitude and climate are homogeneous.

Recording of data

Records of births in Aberdeen are routinely kept on the Aberdeen Maternal and Neonatal Data Bank, which has records stretching back to 1948 (Samphier and Thompson, 1982). All the factors considered below are routinely recorded.

Epoch

It was decided to limit the study to the 23 192 births occurring in the period 1975–1980. There were two reasons for this restriction. First, coding practices were standardised in 1975 and when analysis was started the most recent year for which data was available was 1980; secondly, earlier work (reported in Carr-Hill and Pritchard, 1983, and examined in detail in chapter 2) showed that there has been a secular trend in mean birthweight for gestation at pre-term weeks. To include data over a longer period would, therefore, have introduced the further complexity of allowing for a secular trend.

EXCLUDED PREGNANCY OUTCOMES

Stillbirths

All stillbirths have been excluded from the analysis. The major reason for this lies in a lack of confidence about the relationship between fetal death, delivery and gestation. During this period, there was a hospital stillbirth rate of 9.3 per thousand, and the majority of those were antepartum.

Multiple pregnancy

Multiple pregnancies have been excluded from the sample. Babies of multiple pregnancies are, on average, substantially lighter than singletons and may be thought of as a discrete group of births whose inclusion would affect the results of the survey. Their exclusion means that the assessment is for the normal range of birthweight in singleton pregnancies. During this period there was a hospital multiple pregnancy rate of 12.9 per thousand maternities.

THE DATA AVAILABLE

The population chosen is therefore the 23 192 singleton live births occurring in AMH in the period 1975–1980 for which adequate records were available at the time of analysis. For the purposes of analysis, however, there are some additional restrictions which are described below.

The Data Appendix to this chapter documents the distribution of the variables included in the study for this basic 'reference' population of 23 192: the main 'standards' population of 17 528 births for analysis after taking into account the criteria for inclusion and exclusion discussed in this chapter; and the subpopulation of 4995 births for whom information was available on the mother's mid-term weight as well as her height.

In general, the attempt has been made to minimise the exclusion from the base population made from the survey, on the grounds that minimising exclusions reduces possible bias. The specific exclusions are detailed below.

Birthweight

Birthweight is recorded in grammes to the nearest 10 grammes. The weighting is performed as soon after birth as is conveniently possible by hospital staff. Information was available for all cases. The means and standard deviations in the three populations were 3310.1 and 506.6, 3335.0 and 402.9 and 3296.5 and 493.8 respectively.

Gestation

Gestational age is recorded in weeks completed since the first day of the last menstrual period (LMP).

The major intention of the survey is to provide estimates of the normal range of birthweight for a given gestational age. In common with other surveys, the numbers of births below 32 and above 42 weeks of gestation are such that it is not possible to be confident about estimates for weeks outside that range. Further, since the analysis discusses the appropriate functional form for birthweight by gestation these values represent a disproportionate source of error at the extremes of the range of gestation. For these reasons only births between 32 and 42 weeks have been included. It can be seen that the 'reference' population included 263 cases (1.1%) where the gestation was unknown or fell outside this range.

The distribution of gestations shows that the modal gestational age is 40 weeks in all these populations. Of the gestations between 32 and 42 weeks inclusive, 1008, 672 and 227 occur before 37 weeks in the three populations, that is 4.3%, 3.8% and 4.5% respectively. There is no major difference between the three populations.

Certainty of gestation

An assessment of the certainty of gestation is also made, according to the following criteria:

(1) *Certain* – Gestations are recorded as 'certain' either when the date of the LMP is 'certain' or when the date of LMP is approximate (e.g. because of a long last cycle) but there is corroboratory evidence during pregnancy, e.g. a scan, or after delivery. Certain gestation is taken as having the meaning ± 1 week.

(2) *Approximate* – Gestations are recorded as approximate when the date of LMP is approximate in the absence of other evidence, when the date of the LMP is uncertain but other evidence is available or when the LMP was a pill withdrawal bleed. Approximate gestation is taken as having the meaning ± 2 weeks.

(3) *Uncertain* – Other gestations are recorded as uncertain with the meaning ± 4 weeks.

Seventy cases were not coded and have therefore been excluded.

'Uncertain' and 'approximate' gestations have been excluded from the analysis basically for the reasons discussed in chapter 5. However, whilst the exclusion of the 'uncertain' gestations (7.0%) seems obvious given that the estimate of gestation is ± 4 weeks and given the importance of avoiding the simultaneity implicit in the complex measurement model of chapter 5, there might be some doubt as to whether or not 'approximate' gestations (± 2 weeks) should be excluded or included.

The decision to exclude them was reinforced by the observation that, when birthweight is statistically controlled for gestation, the relationship between birthweight and other variables differs significantly in some cases between those for whom gestation is 'certain' and those for whom gestation is 'approximate'. In particular, the crucial correlation between parity and birthweight was significantly reduced in the 'approximate' group as compared to the 'certain' group.

However, as we discussed at some length in chapter 5, the major reasons for this exclusion are, firstly, that, for the 'approximate' group too, some parameter of fetal size has frequently entered into the estimation of the length of gestation. Secondly, the inclusion of the 'approximate' group would add further to the already considerable imprecision that surrounds the estimate of the length of gestation. Because of the importance of having precise data in order to estimate the model of birthweight for gestation and because of the additional problem of simultaneity they would introduce, it was decided also to exclude cases where the gestation was judged to be approximate. This means excluding a further 3585 cases (15.4%).

The 'standards' sample, then, includes only those births (77.3%) whose gestation was coded as certain. It is further noted that, in some cases, a parameter indirectly or directly related to fetal or baby size such as ultrasonic scan may occasionally have entered into the classification of gestation as 'certain' in the form of corroboratory evidence (see Discussion in chapter 5).

Sex

There were 29 cases in the whole population where the sex of the infant was not recorded. Otherwise, the ratio of boys to girls in the three populations were 1.073, 1.078 and 1.088 respectively.

Parity

Parity is a count of the number of previous pregnancies which ended in a live birth or a stillbirth at 28 weeks gestation or later. This is recorded at the antenatal clinic and, where possible, is confirmed by reference to known previous history. There were no missing data values: 10 439, 7705 and 2543 were primiparae in the three populations; that is, 45.0%, 44.0% and 50.9% respectively. The relative preponderance of primiparae in the 'weights' sample is a consequence of our restriction to women for whom *mid-term* weights are available and the known earlier attendance of primiparae.

Maternal height

Maternal height is routinely recorded in millimetres, although for the purposes of these analyses it has been recoded to the nearest centimetre. In the whole population there were 353 cases (1.6%) for whom information on height was not available. The remainder had a mean height of 159.6 with a standard deviation of 6.4. The mothers in the standard sample had a mean of 159.7 with a standard deviation of 6.2 and the mothers in the 'weights' sample a mean height of 159.6 with a standard deviation of 6.2. There is no discernible difference.

Maternal weight

Mothers-to-be are routinely weighed during antenatal visits, the weights being recorded to the nearest 100 grammes. It has been possible to associate weights with the gestational age at which they were taken for the purposes of this survey. In order to ensure relative homogeneity of the values for maternal weight only maternal weights taken between 18 and 22 weeks gestation have been used in analyses which incorporate maternal weight (see chapter 5, page 50 for a discussion). The empirical effects of the bias introduced by this criterion for inclusion in those analyses (clearly, for example, this group must have attended for antenatal care during the relevant weeks of their pregnancy) are discussed at length in the course of the analysis. The 4995 women for whom mid-term weights were available weighed in at an average of 63.0 kg with a standard deviation of 10.5 kg.

Maternal age

The mother's date of birth is routinely recorded and her age computed in completed years from this information. There were 8 cases in the whole population where the age was not known. Among the whole population there were 9.2% who were teenagers and 4.7% who were 35 years or over, whilst among the standards sample there were 6.7% who were teenagers and 4.7% who were 35 years or over, and among the weights sample there were 7.0% who were teenagers and 4.9% who were 35 years or over.

Pre-eclampsia

Pre-eclampsia is routinely coded in Aberdeen in the following way:

(1) *Mild* — Diastolic blood pressure reading of 90 or more on two consecutive occasions at least 24 h apart; Esbach less than 0.25 g/litre.
(2) *Moderate* — Blood pressure criteria as for 'mild' but Esbach between 0.25 and 2.0 g/litre.
(3) *Severe* — Blood pressure criteria as for 'mild' but Esbach 2.0 g/litre or more.

Among the whole population and the standards sample 4.1% had proteinuric (moderate or severe) pre-eclampsia. However, among the weights sample, 246 (or 4.9%) had pre-eclampsia. The slight increase is probably because there are more primiparae among the weights sample (as explained above).

Diabetes

Although diabetes is recorded as a complication of pregnancy, reliable data only refer to insulin-dependent diabetes. There were 123 overt cases reported in the whole population (0.5%) and similar percentages in the 'standards' and 'weights' samples.

Smoking habits

Maternal smoking habits are recorded at booking as the number of cigarettes smoked per day on the basis of self-reporting. Maternal smoking habits, of course, vary during pregnancy and time of booking may vary with parity and social class. No-one was excluded because the data were unavailable, but it must be emphasised that the number cited is self-reported and liable to all the vagaries consequent upon such a measuring instrument. Given this caveat, and noting that around 60% of each population claimed *not* to have smoked, much of the subsequent analysis is conducted using the dichotomous variable not smoked/ smoked. Nevertheless, it is worth noting that, although about the same proportion of each population claimed to be smoking 30 or more cigarettes per day (around 1.5%), half as many of the 'weights' sample (5.6%) claimed to have been smoking 1–9 cigarettes per day as compared to either the whole population (12.0%) or the 'standards' sample (12.1%).

Social class

Although the woman's own premarital occupation and the current occupation are routinely recorded, for all ensuing analyses, social class refers to the husband's occupation classified according to Registrar General's social class. On this basis, there is a considerable amount of missing data in part because of single mothers: 4131 in the whole population (17.8%), 2756 in the 'standards' sample (15.7%); and 1056 in the 'weights' sample (21.0%). Apart from these missing data, the distributions are approximately 23%: 8%: 29%: 22% as between social classes I and II: IIINM: IIIM: IV and V, respectively, in all three populations.

Civil status

The civil status of the infant is recorded on the basis of the registration of the birth. The woman's date of marriage is also routinely recorded. There were two cases where the civil status of the infant was not recorded. The proportion of illegitimate births in the three populations is 8.6%, 5.3% and 6.8% respectively.

Induction

Induced labours are those where the onset of labour was not spontaneous. They include elective caesarian sections and those labours which were initiated by artificial rupture of the membranes and/or the administration of appropriate drugs. Labours which were of spontaneous onset but were subsequently accelerated and caesarian sections after the onset of labour are classified as non-induced.

The slightly higher proportion of induced labours in the 'weights' sample (42.7%) compared to the 'available population' (40.7%), once again reflects the higher proportion of primiparae.

THE FINAL SAMPLE

It can be seen that with the major exception of maternal mid-term weight, reasonably complete data on the 'normal' and 'intermediate' factors are available for each birth. The treatment of missing data will be reported where appropriate in the ensuing analyses. Note that this sample, in common with the samples used in other birthweight surveys, is not a probability sample.

The basic population, then, comprises all the births taking place in a particular hospital context in a particular period of time. As far as possible in a data set of this size, the accuracy of the data has been assured by routine methods (Samphier and Thompson, 1982). The data collected further include many of the factors which are associated with birthweight and all those commonly used in the analysis of birthweight surveys.

The standards sample, then, consists of the 17 528 live singleton births of 'certain' gestation which took place in AMH during the period between 1975 and 1980. Of these, 4995 mothers were weighed between 18 and 22 weeks gestation.

RECODING VARIABLES

The statistical analyses in the remainder of this monograph are, in the main, parametric – that is, they depend upon distributional properties of the data in order that confidence intervals for the coefficient estimates can be calculated. Many of the variables, in their raw form (as originally coded) have highly skewed distributions and, for others, the raw data cannot be relied upon in the degree of detail with which they were originally recorded. For these reasons the following variables have been recoded for the purposes of this analysis as below:

(1) *Gestation* – recorded as the number of days from date of LMP to date of delivery, recoded in number of completed weeks.
(2) *Parity* – directly recorded, recoded as primiparae/multiparae for most analyses and in four categories, 0/1/2/3+, for others.
(3) *Maternal Age* – calculated as the number of days from dates of mother's birth to date of delivery, recoded as numbers of completed years.
(4) *Maternal Height* – originally recorded in millimetres, rounded to the nearest centimetre for this analysis.
(5) *Smoking Habits* – recorded as the number of cigarettes smoked per day: recoded as 'smokes/does not smoke' for some analyses and into five categories, 0/1–9/10–19/20–29/30+, for others.
(6) *Pre-Eclampsia* – recorded as normotensive; mild, moderate or severe pre-eclampsia recoded as normotensive/non-proteinuric pre-eclampsia/proteinuric-pre-eclampsia, i.e. moderate and severe, are combined.
(7) *Social Class* – coded from the husbands' occupations recorded at the clinics into the Registrar General's social classification (Registrar General, 1981); recoded for the analysis as I and II/IIINM/IIIM/IV and V.

TRANSFORMATIONS

Maternal weight-for-height

The existing set of variables includes two parameters of maternal size: viz. maternal height and maternal (mid-term) weight. As Thomson *et al.* (1968) point out, these are highly correlated which makes the assessment of the independent effects of maternal height and maternal (mid-term) weight upon birthweight awkward (see the Discussion in chapter 3). To get round this problem an index of maternal weight-for-height variable (following the suggestion of Billewicz *et al.*, 1962) has been calculated for those women for whom maternal (mid-term) weights are available (the restriction to mid-term weights was explained above). The index, 'maternal z weight', has been calculated as follows: first, the women have been grouped according to their height and means and standard deviations of the ratio weight/height calculated for each group; then for a woman falling into a given height group, h_i, her maternal z weight is given by:

$$\frac{w_{ij}/h_i - \text{mean}\,(w_i/h_i)}{\text{SD}\,(w_i/h_i)}$$

w_{ij} = mid-term weight of jth woman in height group i

h_i = height group i

The value of this index thus gives the relative position of the woman's own weight for height (her w_{ij}/h_i) within the distribution of w_{ij}/h_i for women of her height group. It would clearly be convenient if such an index were distributed independently of maternal height. In these data the correlation coefficient for these data was 0.0023; the index thus provides a satisfactory means of comparing weight/height, whatever the maternal height.

Standardised birthweight score

Finally, in the course of analysis, it became convenient to derive an index for birthweight after standardising for the 'normal' factors. This index is derived in a similar fashion to the weight-for-height index: first, the births are grouped according to the 'normal' factors — gestation (32, ...42), sex (M:F) and parity (0:1+) — and the means and standard deviations calculated for each group; then for a birth of weight (bwt) falling into a given gestation/sex/parity group (GSP_{ijn}) the standardised birthweight score (SBS_o) is given by

$$SBS_o = \frac{bwt_o - \text{mean}\,(bwt_{ijk})}{\text{SD}\,(bwt_{ijk})}$$

The value of this index thus gives the relative position of the weight of this particular birth within the distribution of birthweights for births falling within that gestation/sex/parity group.

The extent to which this index can be treated as being drawn from a normal distribution — which is both practically and statistically convenient — is discussed at length below (see chapters 8 and 9). It is clearly also important to check that such an index is distributed independently of the three standardising factors — gestation, sex and parity (see chapter 8).

STATISTICAL METHODS

The research problems that are usually addressed using birthweight standards tend to be those which seek to test hypotheses about the association between some factor and the trajectory of fetal growth. Given the multiplicity and complexity of the factors which are believed to influence fetal growth rate, it is frequently desirable to 'control' for the effects of other factors in order to assess the effects of a particular factor. Experimental design is obviously crucial in any such research, but the factors which have been characterised as 'normal' and 'intermediate' are present in every pregnancy and it is thus often appropriate to control for their effects by statistical methods.

For this reason, the argument developed in chapters 7 and 8 is, essentially, statistical. The purpose of this section is to outline the main features of the statistical techniques which are going to be used. This is only meant as a summary to aid the general reader and not as a rigorous exposition.

Bivariate analyses

The preliminary analyses rely upon simple breakdowns of birthweight according to the levels of categorical variables and Pearson correlations of birthweight with metric variables. The use of more complex statistical procedures for examining the whole intercorrelation matrix (for example, factor analysis) is avoided, partly because these are preliminary analyses and partly because *a priori* grouping of the variables in the way argued for in chapter 5 is preferred.

While the use of means, standard deviations and Pearson product moment correlation coefficients in this way may serve to give a general impression of the effects of the variables upon birthweight, the former procedure becomes inordinately complex and data-greedy when several variables are considered at once, and the latter is technically inappropriate for non-metric variables (see, for example, our comment on Dowding in chapter 10). The majority of the analyses make use of analysis of variance.

Analysis of variance

The basis of analysis of variance is to separate that part of the variance in the dependent variable which can be 'explained', by a set of independent variables, from the 'residual' variance, which remains 'unexplained'. Variance is measured in terms of the 'sum of squares' (SS) which is the sum of the squared differences between the value of a particular observation and the mean value for all the observations in that set and is calculated as the sum of squares/degrees of freedom.

In analysis of variance, the total sum of squares is seen as being made up of the sum of squares *between* groups defined by the levels of the independent variable(s) and the sum of squares *within* those groups. The sum of squares between groups is calculated as the difference between the group mean and the grand mean, squared and multiplied by the number of observations in that group and summed for all the groups defined by the independent variable. The sum of squares within groups is the sum of the squared difference between each observation and the group mean summed across all the groups. The sum of squares between is referred to as the 'explained' sum of squares, and the sum of squares within as the 'unexplained' or 'residual'. In simple analysis of variance the sums of squares, degrees of freedom and variance are calculated for all cases and for each of the variables under consideration.

In a simple situation, the effects of one independent variable are the same whatever value is taken by other independent variables. Where this is not the case it is possible to specify the way in which any pair or combination of variable act together (e.g. multiplicatively) and make appropriate estimates. It is also possible in a generalised analysis of variance to calculate an additional contribution of the combined effects of two or more variables without any prior specification. In either of these situations the additional component of the explained sum of squares over and above the separate ('main') effects is referred to as the interaction effect.

Analysis of variance was designed to examine the effects of non-metric, categorical, variables on an independent variable. The effects of metric independent variables are better assessed by regression (see immediately below). In the ensuing analyses both metric independent variables (maternal height and z weight, for example) and non-metric independent variables (sex and parity, for example) are to be considered. To cope with this situation analysis of covariance can be used which takes account of regression effects and the effects of categorical variables in the same analyses.

Multiple regression

In some cases, the ensuing analyses make use of the techniques of multiple regression, either in the context of an analysis of variance or in its own right. It is a technique appropriate for the analyses of the association between metric variables.

In the case of simple regression, where there is only one independent variable, regression estimates the straight line which gives the 'best fit' for the bivariate distribution of the observations. The 'best fit' line is drawn so as to minimise the squared distance of the values of the dependent variable from the regression line: a 'least squares' solution. Once the regression line has been calculated, values of the dependent variable can be predicted from the equation.

$$y = A + B_x$$

where y is the dependent variable, x is the independent variable, A is the point at which the regression line crosses the y axis (the 'intercept'), and B is the slope on the regression line (for each unit increase in x, y will change by B).

In multiple regression (where there is more than one independent variable) the equation has the general form

$$y = A + B_1x_1 + B_2x_2 + B_3x_3$$

The 'best fit' line is, once again, calculated according to the least squares principle.

The method of multiple regression used in this monograph is the 'hierarchical' method. In this method the regression line for each independent variable is calculated sequentially in an order determined, in this case, by the order of priority outlined in chapter 5. The 'effect' of each independent variable is estimated having first removed the effects due to the correlation of independent variables which precede it in the equation (for further details, see Nie *et al.*, 1978, chapter 20).

All the analyses reported have been performed using procedures available in the Statistical Package for the Social Sciences (SPSS) (Nie *et al.*, 1978, 1980) and the reader is referred to their more detailed descriptions. Thus, the majority of the analyses of variance have made use of the **MANOVA** package which provides:

(1) Estimates of the sums of squares accounted for by each of the variables. The extent to which the sum of squares explained might have arisen by chance is assessed using the F ratio, which is defined as the ratio between the variance due to an independent variable and the residual variance, and MANOVA supplies values for the F ratio and the significance of an F test.

(2) Estimates for the effects of a given level of categorical variables and for the slope of the regression line for metric independent variables together with their 't' values and confidence intervals. The convention adopted in the discussion of the analysis is to refer to estimates of particular values of non-metric variables as parameter estimates and to refer to the slopes of regression lines for metric independent variables as coefficients.

The *new regression* package of SPSS has been used for some multiple regression analyses. *New regression* provides (*inter alia*) partial and multiple regression coefficients, partial and multiple correlation coefficients and an analysis of covariance together with the appropriate 'F' ratios and the significance of the 'F' tests.

Statistical tests

There are a number of specific test procedures used in chapters 7 and 8 which should be mentioned.

Testing for values of coefficients and parameters

The task of model building does not end with the estimation of a set of parameters. We have adopted the conventional statistical fiction that this analysis of a population should, for the purposes of drawing inferences about the 'true' value of the parameters, be treated as a sample. We can thus refer the estimates to a theoretical sampling distribution. With the extra assumption that the error terms are drawn from a *normal* sampling distribution, it is possible to refer the 't' values given by MANOVA for each coefficient or parameter estimate to a student '*t*' distribution with $T - K$ degrees of freedom (where T is the number of observations and K is the number of parameters being estimated in the model).

Chow tests for combining subpopulation

At several places in the subsequent text, the question arises as to whether separate coefficients are appropriate for different segments of the population. The appropriate test is a modification of the test for whether a single coefficient is significantly different from zero. Essentially, the situation can be modelled by including slope dummy variables for each of the variables suspected of having different coefficients and a dummy intercept for each subpopulation.

Then the appropriate test is simply the comparison of the reduction in the sum of squared errors obtained by including these variables with the sum of squared errors in the complete model with both the numerator and denominator adjusted by their appropriate degrees of freedom (Hanushek and Jackson, 1977, chapter 5).

Comparing raw standardised scores

One of the purposes of the analytic strategy proposed in chapter 5 is to derive birthweight scores standardised for gestation, sex and parity and, sometimes, for maternal height and z weight as well. This procedure has several advantages for subsequent analysis and especially if the distribution can be treated as approximately normal. There exist several statistics for testing whether or not a departure from normality is significant (for example, tests of skewness and kurtosis vis-a-vis the normal distribution values of 0 and 3 respectively, or a Kolmogorov–Smirnov test for the comparison of an observed and theoretical distribution). However, the interest here is not in whether a particular distribution is significantly different from the normal in the statistical sense, but whether the differences affect the use to which the standardised scores will be put.

The procedure that has been adopted is to examine the slope of the regression line (raw against standardised). If the distribution were normal, then the estimate would be equal to one standard deviation: departures from that value provide a measure of departures from normality.

DATA APPENDIX

This appendix supplements the data description provided in chapter 5. It provides further information about the samples used in the illustrative development of standards (Section 2) and the research chapters (Section 3).

Data are provided on the distribution of the variables which play a part in the analyses presented in the book for three groups:

(1) For the 'basic population' – all singleton live births occurring in the Aberdeen Maternity Hospital from the middle of 1975 up to and including the first six months of 1981, for which adequate records were available at the time of analysis – a total of 23 192 births.

(2) For the 'standards sample' – singleton live births of 'certain' gestation between 32 and 42 weeks where the sex of the infant, maternal parity and maternal height were recorded – a total of 17 528 births.

(3) For the 'weight sample' – a subsample of the standards sample where maternal height was taken between 18 and 22 weeks gestation – a total of 4995 births.

As a preliminary, the distribution over the years is given in table 6.1.

Table 6.1

Year of delivery	Basic population		Standards sample		Weight sample	
	N	%	N	%	N	%
1975*	2273	9.8	1858	10.6	0	0.0
1976	3479	15.0	2478	14.1	2	0.0
1977	3409	14.7	2407	13.7	9	0.0
1978	3734	16.1	2828	16.1	1374	27.5
1979	4082	17.6	3198	18.2	1496	29.9
1980	4267	18.4	3291	18.8	1436	28.7
1981*	1948	8.4	1468	8.4	680	13.6
Total	23 192	100.0	17 528	100.0	4995	100.0

*Part years only.

The order in which the data are presented below follows the presentation in chapter 5.

(a) *Birthweight*

Basic population		Standards sample		Weight sample	
Mean	SD	Mean	SD	Mean	SD
3310.1	506.6	3335.0	402.9	3296.5	493.8
N = 23 176		17 528		4995	

16/23 192 (0.1%) observations in the basic population have missing birthweight data.

(b) *Length of Gestation*

Weeks of gestation	Basic population		Standards sample		Weight sample	
	N	%	N	%	N	%
32	49	0.2	34	0.2	13	0.3
33	95	0.4	62	0.4	22	0.4
34	144	0.6	99	0.6	27	0.5
35	245	1.1	159	0.9	54	1.1
36	475	2.0	318	1.8	111	2.2
37	975	4.2	687	3.9	224	4.5
38	2364	10.2	1791	10.2	563	11.3
39	5293	22.8	4231	24.1	1203	24.1
40	7544	32.5	5916	33.8	1630	32.6
41	4945	21.3	3749	21.4	1013	20.3
42	800	3.4	482	2.7	135	2.7
Other	263	1.1	0	0.0	0	0.0
Total	23 192	100.0	17 528	100.0	4995	100.0

(c) *Certainty of Gestation*

Certain	17 935	77.3
Approximate	3558	15.4
Uncertain	1631	7.0
Uncoded	69	0.3
Total	23 192	100.0

Certain gestations only are used in the standards and maternal weight samples.

(d) *Sex*

	Basic population		Standards sample		Weight sample	
	N	%	N	%	N	%
Boys	11 983	51.7	9091	51.9	2603	52.1
Girls	11 180	48.2	8437	48.1	2392	47.9
Missing	29	0.1	0	0.0	0	0.0
Total	23 192	100.0	17 528	100.0	4995	100.0

(e) *Birth Rank*

(i) *Parity*

	Basic population N	%	Standards sample N	%	Weight sample N	%
0	10 439	45.0	7705	44.0	2543	50.9
1	8575	37.0	6695	38.2	1632	32.7
2	3100	13.4	2338	13.3	613	12.3
3	765	3.3	563	3.2	153	3.1
4	202	0.9	149	0.9	35	0.7
5	70	0.3	46	0.3	12	0.2
6	24	0.1	16	0.1	1	0.0
7	12	0.1	11	0.1	4	0.1
8	3	0.0	2	0.0	0	0.0
9	3	0.0	3	0.0	2	0.0
Missing	0	0.0	0	0.0	0	0.0
Total	23 192	100.0	17 528	100.0	4995	100.0

(ii) *Pregnancy Number*

	Basic population N	%	Standards sample N	%	Weight sample N	%
1	8601	37.1	6356	36.3	2042	40.9
2	8147	35.1	6278	35.8	1619	32.4
3	4040	17.4	3073	17.5	822	16.5
4	1501	6.5	1141	6.5	321	6.4
5	562	2.4	431	2.5	125	2.5
6	193	0.8	145	0.8	39	0.8
7	90	0.4	61	0.3	14	0.3
8	36	0.2	23	0.1	8	0.2
9	14	0.1	12	0.1	3	0.1
10+	5	0.0	5	0.0	1	0.0
Missing	3	0.0	3	0.0	1	0.0
Total	23 192	100.0	17 528	100.0	4995	100.0

(f) *Maternal Height* (cm)

Basic population Mean	SD	Standards sample Mean	SD	Weight sample Mean	SD
159.6	6.4	159.7	6.2	159.6	6.2
N = 22 839		17 528		4995	

353/23 192 (1.6%) observations in the basic population have missing height data.

(g) *Maternal Weight* (0.10 kg units)

Basic population		Standards sample		Weight sample	
Mean	SD	Mean	SD	Mean	SD
629.1	105.8	630.3	104.7	630.3	104.7
N = 6467		4995		4995	

16 725/23 192 (72.5%) observations in the basic population have missing weight data.
12 533/17 528 (71.5%) observations in the standards sample have missing weight data.

(h) *Maternal Age*

	Basic population		Standards sample		Weight sample	
	N	%	N	%	N	%
-19	2140	9.2	1171	6.7	349	7.0
20–24	7759	33.5	5585	31.9	1659	33.1
25–29	8415	36.3	6761	38.6	1810	36.1
30–34	3755	16.2	3138	17.9	928	18.5
35–39	917	4.0	726	4.1	205	4.1
40+	199	0.7	142	0.6	42	0.8
Missing	7	0.0	5	0.0	2	0.0
Total	23 192	100.0	17 528	100.0	4995	100.0

(i) *Pre-eclampsia*

	Basic population		Standards sample		Weight sample	
	N	%	N	%	N	%
None	16 213	69.9	12 195	69.9	3337	66.8
mild	6027	26.0	4613	26.3	1412	28.3
Proteinuric	952	4.1	720	4.1	246	4.9
Total	23 192	100.0	17 528	100.0	4995	100.0

(j) *Maternal Diabetes*

	Basic population		Standards sample		Weight sample	
	N	%	N	%	N	%
None	23 069	99.5	17 431	99.6	4961	99.3
Overt	123	0.5	97	0.4	34	0.7
Total	23 192	100.0	17 528	100.0	4995	100.0

(k) *Smoking* (self-reported cigarettes smoked per day)

	Basic population		Standards sample		Weight sample	
	N	%	N	%	N	%
0	13 340	57.5	10 465	59.7	3084	61.7
1-9	2740	12.0	2128	12.1	275	5.6
10-19	3568	15.4	2529	14.4	804	16.1
20-29	2297	9.9	1521	18.7	518	10.4
30+	361	1.6	226	1.3	91	1.7
N/S	886	3.8	659	3.8	223	4.5
Total	23 192	100.0	17 528	100.0	4995	100.0

(l) *Social Class* (husband's occupation)

	Basic population		Standards sample		Weight sample	
	N	%	N	%	N	%
I and II	5381	23.2	4415	25.2	1136	22.8
IIInm	1757	7.6	1427	8.1	395	7.9
IIIm	6826	29.4	5178	29.5	1352	27.1
IV and V	5097	22.0	3752	21.4	1056	21.0
Missing	4131	17.8	2756	15.7	1056	21.0
Total	23 192	100.0	17 528	100.0	4995	100.0

(m) *Civil Status of Infant*

	Basic population		Standards sample		Weight sample	
	N	%	N	%	N	%
Legitimate	21 196	91.4	16 470	94.0	4654	93.2
Illegitimate	1994	8.6	1058	5.3	341	6.8
Unknown	2	0.0	0	0.0	0	0.0
Total	23 192	100.0	17 528	100.0	4995	100.0

(n) *Induction*

	Basic population		Standards sample		Weight sample	
	N	%	N	%	N	%
Induced	9338	40.7	7195	41.0	2132	42.7
Not induced	13 630	58.8	10 264	58.6	2856	57.2
Missing	107	0.5	69	0.4	7	0.1
Total	23 192	100.0	17 528	100.0	4995	100.0

7

Deriving empirical birthweight standards—1: preliminaries and the functional relation of birthweight to gestation

INTRODUCTION

The general approach to the development of birthweight standards has been discussed in chapter 5 and the material from the Aberdeen Maternity and Neonatal Data Bank has been described in chapter 6. The same two chapters set out the elements of an analytic strategy and the appropriate statistical methods by which research standards controlling for the effects of 'normal' and 'intermediate' factors would be derived. Five stages were proposed: the intention of this and the next chapter is to illustrate this analytic strategy and to show how standards for research can be derived from the available material. The particular issues involved in elaborating standards for clinical use are discussed in more detail in chapter 9.

This and the following chapter are arranged in sections according to the analytic strategy laid out in chapter 5. This chapter is concerned with the first three steps. As a preliminary the next section examines the relationships between birthweight and the other variables considered in this study *via* the correlation matrix. The following two sections discuss the possibility of excluding some variables and reducing the number of levels to be considered. The remainder of this chapter then explores the extent to which it is possible to find a convenient functional form for the relationship between birthweight and gestational age.

The data have been presented and described in chapter 6. The exclusions were dealt with in detail there. The analyses in this chapter are concerned solely with the main standards sample ($N = 17\,528$); the analyses in the next chapter will also consider the weights sample ($N = 4995$).

79

PRELIMINARY ANALYSIS

The purpose here is to:

(1) ascertain whether the population is relatively homogeneous in terms of variables which are not included in the analysis;

(2) note whether there are any 'peculiar' characteristics of the population and account for their peculiarities;

(3) make some preliminary decisions about what variables to incorporate in the analysis and the form they ought to take.

The data are examined with these objectives in mind via an examination of the correlation coefficients between birthweight and those variables which may influence birthweight. Because this is, in a sense, a preliminary exercise, Pearsonian correlation coefficients have been used throughout even though they are not strictly appropriate for those variables measured on a nominal or ordinal scale. The use of more complex statistical procedures such as factor analysis to analyse the whole intercorrelation matrix has been avoided. This is partly because this is only the first stage of the analysis but mostly because the analytic strategy argued for in chapter 5 implies that an *a priori* grouping of variables is to be preferred.

However, because gestation explains so much of the variance in birthweight ($r^2 = 0.187$ in this standards sample) and because the focus of the monograph is on standards of birthweight-for-gestation, there are good grounds for making the check both without controlling for gestation and, through partial correlation, with gestation controlled. In table 7.1 sex and parity are also controlled by dividing the population into sex and parity groups. The criteria used in preparing table 7.1 are that correlation coefficients have been included where $r \geqslant 0.05$ and where the F ratio is significant ($P \leqslant 0.05$), which are liberal criteria given the size of the population being considered.

Examining table 7.1 in terms of the objectives is the preliminary exercise.

Factors not included in the analysis

There are two characteristics of the pregnancy which, both for *a priori* reasons and on the basis of arguments earlier in this monograph, one might have expected to have been included in this analysis. These are 'certainty of gestation' and induction. The former, which is an indication of clinical doubt about the coherence of the estimated gestation and the observed birthweight, has been completely excluded from the analysis for the theoretical reasons discussed in chapter 5. As shown in chapter 2, the latter, which potentially means that labour is brought forward to an earlier point in a postulated fetal growth curve of that baby, might be expected to have a significant effect upon the distribution of birthweight for gestation. Moreover, in this period, about 40% of labours were induced (see Data Appendix of chapter 6) so the numbers affected would not be negligible.

As can be seen from table 7.1, in these data induction has a consistently negative relation to birthweight and, indeed, those induced do have a slightly lower birthweight (by 36 grams) than those not induced. Figure 7.1 shows that

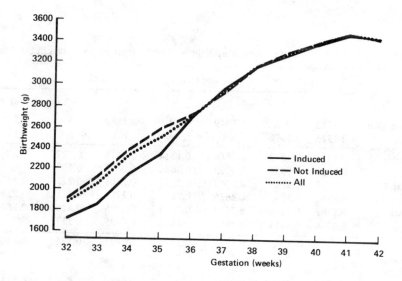

Figure 7.1 Mean birthweight by week of gestation according to whether or not induced

after 35 weeks there is no systematic difference between the birthweights of induced and non-induced babies. However, there is a substantial (*c*. 250 grams) difference between induced and non-induced before 36 weeks.

The results on these particular data set have a very similar pattern to those reported in chapter 2 and thus raise the theoretical problems of 'normality' which were discussed in chapter 5. As we concluded in that discussion, it would be inappropriate to control for induction in deriving standards for pre-term births; for whether or not the baby is induced at any given gestational age, the crucial point is still that it is located at the lower end of an *overall* distribution of birthweight at that gestational age. If, therefore, separate standards were to be derived, this would imply the exclusion of over a quarter of pre-term births, differentially from the lower end of distribution.

The substantial association of induction with birthweight shows how important it is to investigate fully not only the peculiarities of the local population, but also the usual obstetric practices in the area. The issue is discussed further in chapter 12.

Table 7.1 Pearson's product moment correlations of birthweight with variables in the Aberdeen su

	All		Boys		Girls		Para. 0	
	1	2	1	2	1	2	1	
Gestation	0.4323	NA	0.5049	NA	0.4880	NA	0.5317	N
Sex	−0.1323	−0.1570	NA	NA	NA	NA	−0.1352	−0.1
Parity	0.1033	0.1212	0.0886	0.1114	0.1018	0.1275	NA	N
Preg. No.	0.0629	0.0951	0.0593	0.0886	0.0662	0.1039	*	*
Mat. Ht	0.2135	0.2203	0.2043	0.2139	0.2201	0.2256	0.2176	0.2
Mat. Wt	0.2541	0.2844	0.2635	0.2877	0.2798	0.3112	0.2380	0.2
z-wt	0.1989	0.2136	0.2014	0.2232	0.1975	0.2260	0.1819	0.2
Age	0.0704	0.1151	0.0728	0.1183	0.0695	0.1177	*	0.0
Smoking	−0.1487	−0.1763	−0.1717	−0.1714	−0.1873	−0.1984	−0.1443	−0.1
Pre-ec.	*	*	*	*	*	*	*	0.0
Diabet.	*	*	*	*	*	*	*	*
Induct.	−0.0703	*	−0.0920	*	−0.0666	*	−0.1147	*
Soc. Cl.	−0.0693	−0.0649	−0.0738	−0.0718	−0.0599	−0.0647	−0.0544	−0.0

* = does not meet criteria of significance (criteria: $p < 0.05$ and $r > 0.05$).
NA = not applicable.

o order correlations, 2 = partial correlations controlling for gestation

Para. 1+		Boys, 0		Girls, 0		Boys, 1+		Girls, 1+	
	2	1	2	1	2	1	2	1	2
02	NA	0.5466	NA	0.5383	NA	0.4593	NA	0.4763	NA
07	−0.1545	NA	NA	NA	NA	NA	NA	NA	NA
	*	NA	NA	NA	NA	*	*	*	*
	*	*	*	*	*	*	*	*	*
57	0.2176	0.2302	0.2364	0.2081	0.2418	0.2411	0.2297	0.1931	0.2082
89	0.3034	0.2484	0.2743	0.2205	0.2772	0.3198	0.3295	0.2730	0.2967
00	0.2381	0.1996	0.2240	0.1614	0.2053	0.2382	0.2552	0.2096	0.2314
	0.0850	*	0.2240	*	0.0567	*	0.0803	*	0.0842
45	−0.1988	−0.1365	−0.1562	−0.1571	−0.1751	−0.2138	−0.2209	−0.2051	−0.1966
	*	0.0577	0.0644	*	0.0562	*	*	*	*
	*	*	*	*	*	*	*	*	*
33	*	−0.1211	*	−0.1025	*	−0.0535	*	−0.0190	*
14	−0.0821	−0.0511	*	−0.0565	−0.0628	−0.0821	−0.0705	−0.0971	−0.0997

Peculiar characteristics

In general, the effects of the various factors identified as being associated with birthweight are in the direction that would be anticipated from the literature. The notable exceptions are in the cases of pre-eclampsia and maternal diabetes.

Pre-eclampsia

More detailed analysis of the relation between the categories of pre-eclampsia and birthweight shows that the 'peculiar' positive effects of pre-eclampsia occur because of the predominance of 'mild' (non-proteinuric) pre-eclampsia. Thus, whilst the overall mean birthweight is 3335.0 (N = 17 528), the mean birthweight for the 12 195 normotensives (69.6% of the population) is slightly higher at 3340.8 and mean birthweight for the 4613 mild (non-proteinuric) pre-eclamptics (26.3% of the population) is slightly higher again at 3354.5. This distribution, which is partly a result of local diagnostic criteria, accounts for the observed positive correlation: in fact, the effects of moderate and severe pre-eclampsia are in the expected, negative direction (see also chapters 2 and 11).

Maternal diabetes

Similarly, maternal diabetes shows no significant association with birthweight in this population. One explanation is simply that there are very few of them (123) as information on diabetes relates only to established, insulin-dependent diabetics (see chapter 6). At the same time, over the period concerned, these mothers have been the subject of a very active policy of pre-pregnancy counselling, antenatal monitoring and regulation (Sutherland *et al.*, 1970). It may be that the lack of the expected positive correlation between diabetes and birthweight reflect the success of this policy. This is another example of the necessity to take local clinical practice into account.

Preliminary decisions about variables

Because of the 'traditional' use of pregnancy number rather than parity — wherein only live births and stillbirths at or after 28 weeks are counted — in Aberdeen (cf. Thomson *et al.*, 1968), it was felt necessary to make a decision as to which was the most appropriate variable to use for analysis. This is especially important since, in recent years, about 10 per cent of *primiparae* have had a previous pregnancy which ended in a therapeutic abortion (Pritchard and Thompson, 1982).

In table 7.1, both pregnancy number and parity are correlated significantly with birthweight for both boys and girls, but the correlation coefficients for pregnancy number are, in all cases, significantly lower than for parity (using a z test for the difference between two correlation coefficients). Moreover, within any given parity group there is no significant effect upon birthweight due to pregnancy number; whilst there may well be differences, for example between the effects of a preceding spontaneous and therapeutic abortion on birthweight, this does not show up in this cross-sectional analysis. Given, also, that when obstetric history is self-reported, parity is likely to be more accurate, it has been preferred in the subsequent analyses.

DISPENSING WITH VARIABLES

On *a priori* grounds, discussed in chapter 5, the 'normal factors' of gestation and sex are not considered as candidates for removal from analysis. Equally, the 'non-normal' factors (such as social class) only become relevant after standards have been established. This section is therefore concerned only with the 'intermediate' factors.

Of these, the population under consideration does not permit the analysis of the effects of ethnicity. Parity is conventionally included in standards (but note the Swedish practice noted in chapter 5) and is further considered both later in this chapter and in the next chapter. The preliminary analysis showed that both maternal height and maternal z weight were significantly correlated with birthweight in both zero order and partial (gestation controlled) correlations in each of the sex/parity groups. The strength of the associations and their apparent stability provide good grounds for continuing to include these variables in subsequent analyses, and their effects are discussed in detail in the next chapter.

The only potential candidate for exclusion is, therefore, maternal age. In the preliminary correlation analyses maternal age was related positively to birthweight in both sex groups whether or not gestation was controlled. Within parity groups, however, whilst the zero order correlation with birthweight disappeared, the first order correlation of maternal age with birthweight (gestation controlled) remained significant within each of the sex/parity groups. Nevertheless, it was decided to defer consideration of the role of maternal age in a predictive or research model until after the inclusion of the effects of maternal size (see chapter 8).

REDUCING THE NUMBER OF LEVELS

In both the preliminary analysis and in discussing the effects of maternal age, parity has been categorised as 0 or 1+, except when considering the correlations with parity itself. In a sense, therefore, those analyses have presupposed the results of the analysis immediately below for convenience of presentation.

The question at issue is whether reducing the number of levels for parity by combining levels makes any significant difference to the descriptive power of the model derived. The various levels of parity can clearly be combined in many different ways (0; 1; 2; 3; 4+: 0; 1+2; 3: 4+: etc.). Combining them as 0; 1+ (a division between first- and later-born) was the convention adopted by Thomson *et al.* (1968) – and many others – and represents a parsimonious division. The '1+' component of that dichotomy represents parities 1 to 9 in the Aberdeen population, and it would be possible to ask whether parity accounts for a significant proportion of the variance in birthweight among these later born babies.

The answer will depend, of course, on the order in which variables are introduced into the analysis, i.e. on whether variations in parity are seen as having logical precedence over other intermediate factors. The view taken here is that, whilst the division between *primiparae* and *multiparae* is at least as important

Table 7.2   Maternal mid-term weight and maternal z weight by parity

Parity	Maternal mid-term weight				
	In kg			*Standardised for height*	
	Mean	SD	N	Mean	SD
0	62.3	10.0	2543	−0.077	0.927
1	63.1	10.5	1632	0.039	1.000
2	64.5	11.2	613	0.180	1.046
3+	66.3	12.5	207	0.311	1.197
All	63.0	10.5	4995	0.006	0.984

in its own right as other 'intermediate' factors, there are no strong theoretical grounds for supposing that birthweight should increase with higher parity except insofar as babies born to higher parous women tend to be heavier. This apparently paradoxical statement can be understood in the light of table 7.2 which shows that in this population both maternal weight and z weight increase with parity, and we know that birthweight increases with maternal weight (see Billewicz and Thomson, 1973). The analysis, therefore, proceeds, initially, in terms of a 0/1+ dichotomy – returning to the question towards the end of the next chapter.

THE RATE OF CHANGE OF BIRTHWEIGHT BY GESTATION

Introduction

At the outset of this monograph it was suggested that standards were principally used to assess either the intrauterine growth of individual babies (mainly 'clinical' use) or the effects of various factors on that rate of growth (mainly 'research' use). The standards developed in the next chapter refer directly to the distribution of birthweights observed in particular gestation/sex/parity groups in a particular population. These and similar standards can be seen as constituting a statement that, in the particular population from which the standards were derived, babies born at a particular gestation of a particular sex to mothers of a particular parity had, on average, grown in a way such that they had attained a certain weight at birth. The standards are, therefore, essentially *standards of birthweight for gestation rather than standards of fetal growth.*

This empirical approach to the development of standards eschews the use of birthweights to assess a pattern of fetal growth whose form is then used to derive fetal growth standards. As such, it differs from the approach of Thomson *et al.* (1968) or Altman and Coles (1980) which uses smoothed graphs of birthweight by gestation to estimate normal growth. Altman and Coles (1980) appeal to an underlying sense of the statistical neatness of biological phenomena when they comment:

...it is reasonable to assume that, in the population, mean birthweight changes smoothly with increasing gestational age, so irregularities in the observed data may be smoothed out. Similarly, we would expect the amount of variability around these means to change smoothly with gestational age.

The assumption does not, however, seem reasonable. While some babies born at a particular gestation may have followed a similar pattern of growth to that followed by some babies born at other gestational ages, others may not: indeed, the pattern of growth may have affected the gestational age at which birth, whether following a spontaneous or an induced onset of labour, occurred. For a particular gestational age at delivery, babies may have followed very different patterns of growth. The amount of variability about the mean for that gestational age and the mean itself reflect the peculiar combination of patterns of growth of the babies born at that age. The rate of change between mean birthweight at increasing gestational ages does not necessarily provide any information about the pattern of intrauterine growth between gestational ages unless it can be assumed that factors which determine the pattern of fetal growth are *not* determinants of the timing of the onset of labour and that the size of the baby itself does not influence the gestational age at which the baby is born (see also the discussion in chapter 5).

Nevertheless, the subsequent analyses in this chapter make a serious attempt to fit a functional form to the relation between mean birthweight and gestational age. In the first place, as Altman and Coles have amply demonstrated in devising their nomogram (1980), smoothed curves have particular clinical utility and the use of computational algorithms are convenient for the routine recording of standardised birthweights between revisions of the standards. Secondly, it is of interest to compare these 'modern' Aberdeen data with that of Thomson *et al.* (1968) which Altman and Coles (1980) re-analysed (see below). Finally, detailed analysis of the rate of change of mean birthweight may clarify some of the issues in the arguments above and in chapter 5.

Fitting birthweight to gestation

Although simple inspection of the increments associated with increasing gestational age would suggest that they are not uniform over the range of gestations considered, an initial sense of the effects of increasing gestational age may be gained by examining the linear regression of birthweight on gestation. Table 7.3 shows the regression for each of the four sex/parity groups. The pair of coefficients for the boys are similar, but larger than the pair of coefficients for the girls; while the constants are larger for first born than for later born and the constant for the girls is markedly less than that for the boys. Clearly different models are required for the four sex/parity groups.

Table 7.3 also shows the mean of the values estimated from the regression equation and the observed means for each week of gestation. Before the 38th week of gestation, the estimated means are consistently larger than the observed means, as are the estimates for the 41st and 42nd gestational weeks. The discrepancies for the weeks between 37 and 41 tend to be markedly smaller than the discrepancies in the earlier ('pre-term') weeks and for week 42. The decrease in mean birthweight between 41 and 42 weeks is a problematic feature of all the observed distributions.

The question is whether a more appropriate model and/or a better fit can be found. The regression method, of course, is such that a closer fit would be anticipated to those gestational weeks where the number of observations is largest. However, the consistency of the pattern of the residuals would suggest either that a different functional form, giving a greater increment in the early weeks than in the later — or a mix of two functional forms — might more appropriately represent a postulated fetal growth process as well as providing a closer fit to the data. Alternatively, separate models estimated for pre-term and term births, whilst not pretending to represent a fetal growth process, may well provide a closer fit to the data. These possibilities are considered in turn below.

Different functional forms

Table 7.4 shows that a logistic form $[\log (p/1 - p)]$ which is one of the family of growth curves and, especially, a quadratic form (gestation^2 + gestation) account for more of the total sum of squares than the linear model. The considerably greater reduction using the quadratic form is statistically highly significant using an ordinary F test for non-zero coefficients (for example, for boys para 0, $F = 84.2, p < 0.001$). It is important to stress, however, that this does not imply anything more than that the statistical model is providing a better fit to the data: in particular, there can be no implication that there is a *quadratic fetal growth process.*

The pattern of residuals for the logistic curve was very similar to those observed with the linear model. Inspection of the residuals for the quadratic form (table 7.5) shows how close the fit is for the gestations between 38 and 41 weeks where, admittedly, the numbers are largest. For the earlier weeks of gesta-

Table 7.3 Regression equation (constant and coefficient) for linear regression of birthweight on gestation and the observed and predicted means and raw residual by gestation

Constant coefficient	Boys, para 0 −2500.11 147.53			Girls, para 0 −2509.03 144.32			Boys, para 1+ −2411.68 148.46			Girls, para 1+ −2314.81 142.51		
	Obs. mean	Est. mean	Resid.	Obs. mean	Est. mean	Resid.	Obs. mean	Est. mean	Resid.	Obs. mean	Est. mean	Resid.
32 weeks	1843.08	2220.94	−377.86	1790.00	2109.09	−319.09	1970.00	2339.18	−369.18	1902.50	2245.81	−343.31
33 weeks	2134.62	2368.47	−233.86	1976.47	2253.40	−276.93	2176.11	2487.65	−311.54	1926.47	2388.33	−461.86
34 weeks	2339.12	2516.01	−176.89	2133.81	2397.72	−263.91	2338.97	2636.11	−247.15	2282.11	2530.85	−248.75
35 weeks	2489.77	2663.54	−173.77	2314.12	2542.04	−227.92	2582.77	2784.58	−201.81	2504.86	2673.37	−168.51
36 weeks	2701.17	2811.07	−109.90	2661.20	2686.35	−25.15	2836.82	2933.04	−96.22	2639.67	2815.89	−176.22
37 weeks	2924.18	2958.60	−34.42	2778.76	2830.67	−51.91	3047.89	3081.51	−33.62	2953.47	2958.41	−4.94
38 weeks	3176.96	3106.14	70.82	3021.41	2974.98	46.42	3304.58	3229.58	74.61	3140.68	3100.93	39.75
39 weeks	3302.06	3253.67	48.39	3166.42	3119.30	47.12	3396.64	3378.43	18.20	3292.20	3243.45	48.75
40 weeks	3420.48	3401.20	19.28	3287.46	3263.62	23.84	3546.02	3526.90	19.12	3405.58	3385.97	19.60
41 weeks	3506.03	3548.73	−42.70	3377.18	3407.93	−30.75	3646.53	3675.36	−28.83	3483.74	3528.49	−44.75
42 weeks	3472.95	3696.27	−223.32	3313.07	3552.25	−239.18	3570.99	3823.83	−252.84	3469.10	3671.01	−201.91

Table 7.4 Analysis of variance for the regression of birthweight on different functional forms of gestation

		$SS_{resid.}$	$SS_{gest.}$	$F_{gest.}$
a. Boys para 0	Linear	717083034	202196527	1118.86
	Log	713279209	206000351	1145.99
	Gest² ⎱	702173957	⎰197951834	1118.35
	Gest ⎰		⎱ 19153770	108.21
b. Girls para 0	Linear	652789210	175867163	1015.13
	Log	649470596	179185777	1039.57
	Gest² ⎱	639270635	⎰172180635	1014.60
	Gest ⎰		⎱ 17205127	101.38
c. Boys para 1+	Linear	985740417	227570972	1192.18
	Log	981911380	231400009	1216.96
	Gest² ⎱	970564348	⎰223 28460	1188.01
	Gest ⎰		⎱ 19 18581	103.30
d. Girls para 1+	Linear	860421058	190 57377	1039.60
	Log	856383873	194 94762	1066.65
	Gest² ⎱	842149882	⎰185 88754	1037.55
	Gest ⎰		⎱22639998	126.30

tion, the patterning of the residuals for the boys is similar, the estimates being lighter than the observed for the first three weeks and heavier for weeks 35 to 37. No such clear pattern is apparent for the girls. The regression equation for girls para 1+ differs considerably from the equations for the other sex/parity groups. The decrease in mean birthweight between 41 and 42 weeks remains problematic.

The findings for the whole range of gestational ages using different functional forms for gestation suggest that different models might be an appropriate way of coping with the different increments in birthweight for increasing gestation among pre-term and term babies. Although it is not certain whether a division at 36 or 37 weeks would provide the best account of the data, the usual clinical division between pre-term ($\leqslant$ 36 weeks) and term ($\geqslant$ 37 weeks) provides a convenient starting point.

Separate models for pre-term and term

Table 7.6 shows the breakdown of the sums of squares for the different functional forms of gestation for 'term' babies (37 to 41 weeks). Once again, the quadratic form 'explains' more of the variance than either the linear or log forms, although for boys para 1+ the reduction in the residual sum of squares is only just significant at the 1% level ($F = 6.91$).

Table 7.7 shows the difference between observed and estimated means for the quadratic form for babies from 37 to 41 weeks. With the exception of girls para 1+, the regression provides a consistent over-estimate for 37 weeks and a

Table 7.5 Regression equation (constant and coefficient) for the regression of birthweight on gestation² + gestation and the observed and predicted means and raw residuals by gestation

	Boys, para 0 −23 534.51			Girls, para 0 −24 006.20			Boys, para 1+ −24 087.97			Girls, para 1+ −26 420.84		
Constant												
coefficient												
g^2	−14.33			−14.55			−14.60			−16.22		
g	1246.88			1264.26			1274.66			1394.39		
	Obs. mean	Est. mean	Resid.	Obs. mean	Est. mean	Resid.	Obs. mean	Est. mean	Resid.	Obs. mean	Est. mean	Resid.
32 weeks	1843.07	1692.76	150.31	1790.00	1547.90	242.10	1970.00	1750.47	219.53	1902.50	1588.88	313.61
33 weeks	2134.62	2008.26	126.35	1976.47	1866.21	110.26	2176.11	2076.11	100.00	1926.47	1928.88	− 2.41
34 weeks	2339.12	2295.11	44.01	2133.81	2155.42	− 21.61	2388.97	2372.55	16.42	2282.11	2236.43	45.66
35 weeks	2489.77	2553.29	− 63.52	2314.12	2415.53	−101.41	2582.77	2639.79	− 57.02	2504.86	2511.55	6.69
36 weeks	2701.17	2782.81	− 81.65	2661.20	2646.52	14.68	2836.82	2877.83	− 41.01	2639.67	2754.22	−114.55
37 weeks	2924.18	2983.68	− 59.51	2778.76	2848.42	− 69.66	3047.89	3086.67	− 38.78	2953.47	2964.45	− 10.97
38 weeks	3176.96	3155.89	21.07	3021.41	3021.20	0.21	3304.58	3266.31	38.37	3140.68	3142.23	− 1.55
39 weeks	3302.06	3299.45	2.62	3166.42	3164.88	1.54	3396.64	3416.75	− 20.11	3292.20	3287.57	4.62
40 weeks	3420.49	3414.34	6.14	3287.46	3279.46	8.00	3546.02	3537.99	8.03	3405.57	3400.47	5.10
41 weeks	3506.03	3500.58	5.45	3377.18	3364.92	12.25	3646.53	3630.02	16.51	3483.74	3480.93	2.81
42 weeks	3472.95	3558.16	− 85.21	3313.07	3421.28	−108.21	3570.99	3692.86	−121.87	3469.10	3528.94	59.86

Table 7.6 Analysis of variance for the regression of birthweight on different functional forms of gestation for 'term' (37 to 41 weeks) babies

		$SS_{resid.}$	$SS_{gest.}$	$F_{gest.}$
Boys para 0	Linear	646596951	68461868	389.11
	Log	646156078	68902739	391.88
	Quad Gest^2	643764314	67992253	388.04
	Gest		3302251	18.85
Girls para 0	Linear	582234449	68546925	410.06
	Log	581803721	68978103	412.94
	Quad Gest^2	579507901	68086554	409.10
	Gest		3186921	19.15
Boys para 1+	Linear	916284547	97804728	518.76
	Log	915951850	98137424	520.71
	Quad Gest^2	915059303	97427617	517.34
	Gest		1602354	8.51
Girls para 1+	Linear	788448529	73064317	408.57
	Log	788011707	73501139	411.25
	Quad Gest^2	785744728	72594630	407.25
	Gest		3173487	17.80

Table 7.7 Observed means – means estimated from the regression of birthweight on the quadratic form of gestation by week of gestation for 'term' (37 to 41 weeks) babies

	Boys, para 0	*Girls, para 0*	*Boys, para 1+*	*Girls, para 1+*
37 weeks	−27.88	−20.01	−39.90	−0.12
38 weeks	27.64	17.90	42.16	−0.27
39 weeks	−4.69	−1.24	−17.08	0.46
40 weeks	−3.88	−3.76	4.34	−0.35
41 weeks	3.87	2.99	0.23	0.20

consistent under-estimate for 38 weeks. The consistency of this pattern, even though the actual value of the discrepancy is small, suggests that the *inclusion* of 37 weeks adversely affects the fit. Table 7.8 also shows the 'observed minus estimated' means for the regression of birthweight on the quadratic form of gestation for term babies but when babies born at 37 weeks are *excluded*. In comparison with the size of the discrepancies noted when babies born at 37 weeks were *included*, the differences between observed and estimated means have been substantially reduced for babies born at 38 or 39 weeks, except for girls para 1+ where there is a very slight increase. The discrepancies are also reduced for para 0 babies at 40 and 41 weeks, although there is an increase for para 1+ babies, particularly para 1+ boys, for those weeks. In general, however,

Table 7.8 Observed means – means estimated from the regression of birthweight on the quadratic form of gestation by week of gestation for babies 38 to 41 weeks gestation

	Boys, para 0	Girls, para 0	Boys, para 1+	Girls, para 1+
38 weeks	3.27	0.97	12.81	−0.36
39 weeks	−4.28	−1.21	−15.90	0.47
40 weeks	2.87	0.78	12.92	−0.33
41 weeks	−1.50	−0.39	−6.90	0.18

the exclusion of 37 week babies from the 'term' group has the effect of making the estimates derived from the regression of birthweight on gestation predict the observed means more accurately when using the quadratic functional form.

Turning to the 'pre-term' group, although the quadratic form of gestation explains more of the total sums of squares than the other functional forms, the difference is never great whether 'pre-term' is defined as 32 to 36 weeks or as 32 to 37 weeks. Moreover, when the 'explained' sums of squares are partitioned for the quadratic form, the 'gestation' element of the equation never explains a significant proportion of the sums of squares in its own right.

Table 7.9 shows the discrepancy between observed and estimated means for each gestational week for the different functional forms of gestation. The different functional forms give broadly similar estimates, although the estimates for girls at 36 and 37 weeks are markedly better when derived from the quadratic rather than from the other functional forms. In general, comparison of the accuracy of the estimates using the definition 32 to 36 weeks and 32 to 37 weeks shows that either gives an equally inaccurate estimate of mean birthweight. Given the numbers of cases at each gestational week, it would be anticipated that the estimate for 36 weeks would be consistently worse when the 37th week is included, and this is the case, particularly for the girls. While the estimate for the 37 week girls para 1+ is less accurate than that when the 37 week is included in the 'term' group (see tables 7.7 and 7.8) the discrepancy is not large and the estimate is improved for the other sex/parity groups. Comparison with the discrepancies between observed and estimated means for the linear form of gestation for weeks 32 to 37 and those derived from the quadratic form of gestation for the whole population (table 7.6) shows that the estimates are consistently more accurate for boys and less accurate for girls para 0 at 34 and 36 weeks and for girls para 1+ at 33, 35 and 37 weeks.

Summary

A number of attempts have been made to discover whether or not it is possible to fit the raw data on birthweight with some function of gestational age so as to provide a good (in the sense of predictively accurate) estimate of mean birthweight by gestation. The results can be summarised as follows. For the popu-

Table 7.9 Observed − expected means derived from the regression of birthweight on gestation for different functional forms of gestation by week of gestation for 'preterm' babies defined (a) 32–36 weeks, (b) 32–37 weeks

Boys para 0

	Linear a	Linear b	Log a	Log b	Quad a	Quad b
32 weeks	−58.99	−47.55	−47.96	−23.39	−23.42	−44.95
33 weeks	31.96	38.10	31.78	42.40	30.88	38.71
34 weeks	35.88	36.71	30.81	31.78	18.30	36.12
35 weeks	−14.05	−18.53	−18.05	−26.45	−27.98	−19.55
36 weeks	−3.25	−13.03	−0.05	−18.05	6.65	−13.70
37 weeks	—	4.08	—	7.52	—	4.52

Boys, para 1+

	Linear a	Linear b	Log a	Log b	Quad a	Quad b
32 weeks	24.38	23.98	39.41	50.59	−19.18	4.79
33 weeks	9.93	9.70	11.74	18.02	3.17	3.21
34 weeks	2.23	2.16	−2.21	0.57	13.94	3.74
35 weeks	−24.53	−24.43	−28.64	−31.51	−12.68	−19.41
36 weeks	8.95	9.22	11.39	4.12	2.62	13.04
37 weeks	—	0.10	—	2.77	—	2.12

Girls para 0

	Linear a	Linear b	Log a	Log b	Quad a	Quad b
32 weeks	81.26	28.09	92.46	49.43	−47.21	53.59
33 weeks	36.97	7.25	35.62	12.40	35.42	13.81
34 weeks	−36.45	−42.72	−43.08	−47.09	21.88	−47.76
35 weeks	−86.91	−69.72	−91.97	−77.32	−35.73	−79.01
36 weeks	29.42	70.06	32.37	65.15	6.40	63.85
37 weeks	—	−19.70	—	−16.30	—	−15.47

Girls, para 1+

	Linear a	Linear b	Log a	Log b	Quad a	Quad b
32 weeks	71.08	129.78	83.10	152.42	110.74	55.37
33 weeks	−111.53	−78.95	−111.39	−74.24	−111.39	−98.37
34 weeks	37.53	43.99	32.31	38.24	19.22	58.48
35 weeks	53.71	34.06	49.28	24.89	38.02	61.38
36 weeks	−18.06	−63.83	−15.90	69.75	−10.05	−44.75
37 weeks	—	17.28	—	20.88	—	7.05

lation as a whole, divided into sex/parity groups, the quadratic form of gestation provided estimates which were markedly more accurate than other functional forms. The decrement in mean birthweight associated with the increase of gestation from 41 to 42 weeks was not, however, fitted by any of the functional forms. The fit could be further improved if the population was divided into those with gestations up to the 37th week and gestations between 38 and 41 weeks (rather than the conventional division at 36 weeks between pre-term and term).

In general, the estimates of mean birthweight derived from the regression of birthweight on gestation are less accurate for girls than for boys and for earlier rather than for later weeks of gestation. When the division after 37 weeks is made, the discrepancies between observed and estimated no longer show consistent patterns across the sex/parity groups. Table 7.10 shows the components

Table 7.10 Regression equations for 'pre-term' and 'term' sex/parity groups

'Pre-term' (weeks 32–37)

	Constant	Gestation
Boys, para 0	−4697.99	205.89
Girls, para 0	−4871.98	207.31
Boys, para 1+	−5106.59	220.39
Girls, para 1+	−5673.50	232.69

'Term' (weeks 38–41)

	Constant	Gestation	Gestation^2
Boys, para 0	−17 700.98	955.33	−10.6842
Girls, para 0	−23 435.90	1231.16	−14.0775
Boys, para 1+	−1458.21	129.12	− 0.1084
Girls, para 1+	−29 644.62	1556.61	−18.2587

of the regression equations for the sex/parity groups for all gestations (excluding week 42), the gestations being divided at 37/38 weeks with a linear form to 37 weeks and a quadratic form for the weeks 38 to 41.

Discussion

The main motivation for this prolonged exercise in curve fitting was the hope that a formula could be devised from which a standardised birthweight score could be computed for routine purposes which would have a clinical and research utility. At first sight, whether the division between 'pre-term' babies and 'term' babies is used or not, for babies born between 38 and 41 weeks gestation the quadratic equations provide very close estimates of mean birthweight for the gestation/sex/parity cells. On the other hand, the discrepancy between observed and estimated means in the weeks up to the 37th week of gestation are relatively large and suggest that the estimates derived from the statistical models would need to be treated with some caution as a basis for clinical decisions in the early weeks. Moreover, whether or not a division between pre-term and term is employed and however it is done there remains an unresolvable discrepancy at 42 weeks.

Overall, however adroit the statistical manipulations, the discrepancies in the earlier gestational weeks are still clinically significant and the computational advantage of the smoothing procedure is lost. Inasmuch as standardised birthweight scores are intended to reflect the distribution in a particular population rather than a hypothetical model of fetal growth, then the curve fitting exercise was a failure. Whilst closer fits could be obtained with a higher order polynomial, there rapidly comes a point when one says that the algebraic complexity involved is less convenient than simply acknowledging that the birthweight distributions for the four sex/parity groups are different within each gestational age. This is the position adopted here and forms the basis of the argument in the next chapter.

Comparison with previous Aberdeen standards

A subsidiary interest was to compare the distributions in these data with an earlier Aberdeen population (reported in Thomson *et al.*, 1968) which subsequently formed the basis of the (widely used) nomograms proposed by Altman and Coles (1980). Table 7.11 compares their formulae with the formulae for the quadratic forms derived on the basis of the more recent Aberdeen populations (including week 42). Their similarity is all the more striking since Altman and Coles (appropriately) made no allowance for the sample sizes in deriving their

Table 7.11 Comparison of the components of the equation for the regression of birthweight (kg) on gestation^2 + gestation from Altman and Coles (1980, p. 43) and those for the Aberdeen population 1975–80 (cf. table 7.5)

		Constant	Gestation	Gestation^2
Boys para 0	A.C.	−22.568	+1.2006	−0.01380
	Study	−23.535	+1.2469	−0.01433
Girls para 0	A.C.	−22.693	+1.2122	−0.01410
	Study	−24.006	+1.2642	−0.01455
Boys para 1+	A.C.	−20.887	+1.1276	−0.01295
	Study	−24.088	+1.2747	−0.01460
Girls para 1+	A.C.	−22.192	+1.2017	−0.01408
	Study	−26.421	+1.3944	−0.01622

equations, while the distribution of the gestational ages assumes considerable importance in the derivation of the equations for the recent population.

The effects of the differences may be gauged by comparing Thomson *et al.*'s median values, estimates derived from Altman and Coles' polynomial regression, and the observed and estimated means for the current population (see table 7.12). One effect of the differences in the equations is that estimates derived from Altman and Coles' equations are larger than those for the recent population in the early gestational weeks, correspond relatively closely over the main (38–41) weeks of gestation and provide a better prediction for the corresponding mean birthweight at 42 weeks. Curiously, the use of the Altman–Coles formulae would provide more accurate estimates of mean birthweight for 32 weeks gestation in the current population. However, since the mean birthweights in gestation/sex/parity cells in the more recent Aberdeen population tend to be lighter than the medians reported by Thomson *et al.*, especially in the early gestational weeks, this means that the use of Altman–Coles formulae for the current population would result in a greater discrepancy between observed and estimated values (see the discussion in chapter 9).

The equations do, therefore, differ. While the differences in the constants of the equations reflects the differences in mean birthweight between the two populations the equations also reflect the differences in the increments associated with increasing gestational age. In general, the more recent population shows smaller increments with increasing gestational age before 37 weeks than the earlier population and somewhat larger thereafter (see the discussion in chapter 2).

Models of birthweight for gestation and fetal growth

The theoretical problem remains: can these various estimates, in practice, be treated as parameters of a structural model relating birthweight, fetal growth and gestational age. Let us suspend, for the moment, our disbelief in such a model because of the serious problems with such a formulation discussed in chapter 5. Then, the analysis presented in the latter part of this chapter could be taken to suggest a pattern of fetal growth in which, between weeks 32 and 38, fetal growth proceeds at a rate between 200 and 235 grams per week. The rate would be faster for girls than for boys and faster for multiparae than for primiparae. From the 38th week on, the rate of growth would be seen as slowing down with increasing gestation, although growth would continue faster for first born girls than for first born boys and, overall, for multiparae than for primiparae.

As an account of growth, this does not seem unreasonable and would lead to the interesting suggestion that sex differences in birthweight are determined prior to 32 weeks gestation and the increment associated with increased parity is related to differences in the growth rate in the last trimester of pregnancy.

Whilst the results of the curve-fitting exercise can be interpreted in this way,

Table 7.12 Comparison of Thomson *et al.* (1968) and Altman and Coles (1980) analysis of data from Aberdeen births 1948–64 with the analysis of more recent (1975–1980) Aberdeen data

| | | Aberdeen 1948-64 | | | Aberdeen 1975-1980 (cf. table 7.5) | | |
		a TBH median	b A.C. poly.	a − b	c Observed mean	d Estimated poly.	c − d
Boys para 0	32 weeks	1.83	1.87	−0.04	1.84	1.69	0.15
	33 weeks	2.01	2.16	−0.15	2.13	2.01	0.12
	34 weeks	2.45	2.42	0.03	2.34	2.30	0.04
	35 weeks	2.66	2.66	0.00	2.49	2.55	−0.06
	36 weeks	2.83	2.86	−0.03	2.70	2.79	−0.08
	37 weeks	3.02	3.04	−0.02	2.92	2.98	−0.06
	38 weeks	3.20	3.19	0.01	3.18	3.16	0.02
	39 weeks	3.29	3.32	−0.03	3.30	3.30	0.00
	40 weeks	3.42	3.41	0.01	3.42	3.41	0.01
	41 weeks	3.46	3.48	−0.02	3.51	3.50	0.01
	42 weeks	3.53	3.52	0.01	3.47	3.56	−0.09
Girls para 0	32 weeks	1.84	1.81	0.03	1.79	1.55	0.24
	33 weeks	2.13	2.09	0.04	1.98	1.87	0.11
	34 weeks	2.32	2.34	−0.02	2.13	2.16	−0.02
	35 weeks	2.56	2.57	−0.01	2.31	2.42	−0.11
	36 weeks	2.80	2.77	0.03	2.66	2.65	0.01
	37 weeks	2.93	2.93	0.00	2.78	2.85	−0.07
	38 weeks	3.06	3.07	−0.01	3.02	3.02	0.00
	39 weeks	3.18	3.19	−0.01	3.17	3.16	0.01
	40 weeks	3.28	3.27	0.01	3.29	3.28	0.01
	41 weeks	3.37	3.33	0.04	3.37	3.36	0.01
	42 weeks	3.32	3.35	0.03	3.31	3.42	−0.11
Boys para 1+	32 weeks	2.08	2.08	0.00	1.97	1.75	0.22
	33 weeks	2.21	2.36	−0.15	2.18	2.08	0.10
	34 weeks	2.63	2.60	0.03	2.39	2.37	0.02
	35 weeks	2.87	2.82	0.05	2.58	2.63	−0.05
	36 weeks	3.01	3.02	−0.01	2.84	2.88	−0.04
	37 weeks	3.17	3.19	−0.02	3.05	3.09	−0.04
	38 weeks	3.30	3.33	−0.03	3.30	3.27	0.03
	39 weeks	3.43	3.45	−0.02	3.40	3.42	−0.02
	40 weeks	3.56	3.54	0.02	3.55	3.54	0.01
	41 weeks	3.63	3.61	0.02	3.65	3.63	0.02
	42 weeks	3.62	3.65	−0.03	3.57	3.69	−0.12
Girls para 1+	32 weeks	1.90	1.99	0.09	1.90	1.59	0.31
	33 weeks	2.24	2.27	−0.03	1.93	1.93	0.00
	34 weeks	2.55	2.51	0.04	2.28	2.24	0.04
	35 weeks	2.67	2.73	−0.06	2.50	2.51	−0.01
	36 weeks	2.93	2.92	0.01	2.64	2.75	−0.11
	37 weeks	3.05	3.08	−0.03	2.95	2.96	−0.01
	38 weeks	3.16	3.21	−0.05	3.14	3.14	0.00
	39 weeks	3.29	3.31	−0.02	3.29	3.29	0.00
	40 weeks	3.38	3.39	−0.01	3.41	3.40	0.01
	41 weeks	3.46	3.43	0.03	3.48	3.48	0.00
	42 weeks	3.42	3.45	−0.03	3.47	3.53	−0.06

such a story would also have to account for the lower proportion of the variance explained by the regression of birthweight on gestation for the earlier weeks, and the size of the errors in the estimates at those weeks. An alternative explanation of all these results is simply that the distribution of birthweight in the earlier gestational weeks reflects a greater heterogeneity in the fetal growth of babies born 'pre-term' than is the case for those born 'at term' (cf. chapter 2 and see chapter 12).

Obviously, the mere fact that mean birthweight increases with increasing gestational age prior to the 42nd week suggests a growth process. Equally obviously, the birthweight of an individual baby is a measure of its intrauterine growth. However, this does not mean that a 'normal' pattern of fetal growth can be estimated from data on observed birthweights at different gestational ages. Indeed, there is an obvious circularity in justifying a description of mean birthweight by gestational age in terms of statistical ('growth') models at the same time as accounting for any discrepancies between the description and the data by the statistical properties of growth curves. This circularity cannot be circumvented by some kind of smoothing procedure but only by having some *a priori* evidence about intrauterine growth.

These conclusions are inconvenient. It would have been useful for clinical purposes if *one* of these simple functional forms had fitted the data. This is partly because the resulting standards then become easier to manipulate (*vide* Altman and Coles nomograms). But the main reason is that, even with fairly large numbers of births in a survey, some gestation/sex/parity cells contain only small numbers. The estimation of an appropriate 'norm' for those cells by extrapolation would be one way of deriving more robust clinical standards for the assessment of future births. Nevertheless, since the meaning of the estimates derived statistically would be dubious, the advantages of using a smoothing procedure for clinical standards are unclear. Empirically derived standards, which have a clearly descriptive status, also have their problems (because, for example, they use retrospective data for the assessment of future births). Nevertheless, given the multitude of problems discussed in this chapter, we prefer the transparency of empirical standards as compared to those derived from a statistical or a doubtful theoretical model.

8
Deriving empirical birthweight standards—2: standardising for normal and intermediate factors

INTRODUCTION: THE RESEARCH STANDARDS FOR GESTATION, SEX AND PARITY

The grounds for attempting to fit a functional form to the relationship of birthweight to gestation in the previous chapter were that it would be computationally convenient and clinically simple, whilst still providing a good representation of the data. However, the most successful of the several attempts implied a separate fit for the 4 sex-parity groups divided between 'term' and 'pre-term' babies; and even so there were *lacunae* among the very early (32 weeks) and very late (42 weeks) gestations. The discussion, therefore, concluded that they are neither computationally convenient nor clinically simple. Moreover, such a set of smoothed relationships would impede the investigation of the birthweight-for-gestation distributions (see chapter 5).

Instead, the procedure adopted at this stage is simply to describe the distribution of birthweights in each of the 44 gestation/sex/parity cells (11 weeks of gestation, 4 sex/parity groups) in terms of its mean and standard deviation (see table 8.1). Whilst this may appear a little more cumbersome, it has the crucial advantage of retaining information on the variability of the distribution. In this way, an individual observation can be located on the distribution of birthweights in the appropriate sex/parity cell by its 'standard deviation score'. For example, a para 0 boy born at 39 weeks weighing 3200 grams would be referred to a distribution with a mean of 3302.6 and a standard deviation of 428.8 (see table 8.1). Its standard deviation score would, therefore, be $(3200 - 3302.6)/428.8 = -0.24$.

This standardised birthweight score has many convenient properties. In the first place, birthweight scores can more easily be compared across gestation, sex and parity groups. In the second place, the mean and standard deviation of a standard deviation score are 0 and 1 respectively which facilitates the inter-

Table 8.1 Means and standard deviations of birthweight in gestation/sex/parity (0, 1+) cells

Week gest.	Boys, parity 0			Girls, parity 0			Boys, parity 1+			Girls, parity 1+		
	Mean	SD	N	Mean	SD	N	Mean	SD	N	Mean	SD	N
32	1843.1	321.8	13	1790.0	496.2	8	1970.0	351.3	5	1902.5	289.7	8
33	2134.6	340.1	13	1976.5	461.5	17	2126.9	339.9	16	1970.6	301.8	16
34	2360.3	502.1	32	2133.8	369.5	21	2382.9	277.6	28	2353.3	408.7	18
35	2489.8	440.2	44	2314.1	443.9	34	2590.0	382.7	46	2550.9	465.3	35
36	2701.2	431.2	77	2657.3	384.4	82	2843.5	440.8	84	2640.2	418.6	75
37	2927.9	435.9	169	2731.0	434.7	143	3045.8	500.8	200	2961.9	437.6	175
38	3177.5	402.5	392	3021.8	412.9	346	3308.8	420.6	562	3141.4	392.2	491
39	3302.6	428.8	901	3165.1	420.8	832	3397.8	435.1	1360	3292.6	419.9	1138
40	3420.5	414.4	1345	3287.9	399.8	1286	3546.3	424.8	1677	3406.6	422.8	1608
41	3508.2	416.3	854	3379.6	393.6	864	3647.4	436.6	1045	3484.3	431.7	986
42	3475.0	454.8	111	3340.5	398.4	121	3570.9	461.3	117	3469.1	437.4	133

pretation both of the estimates of coefficients and of parameters in regression analysis (as $b = \beta$), and of the sums of squares (as the total sum of squares $= N$).

Note that these standardised birthweight scores are *not* in the same form as those proposed by Thomson *et al.* (1968) or Altman and Coles (1980). The former expressed birthweights are centile scores and the standardised scores proposed by the latter had means of 100 and standard deviations of 10. We stress the point here only because our readers are probably accustomed to thinking in terms of centiles or of scores near 100.

It would be even more convenient – that word again! – for clinical purposes if this standardised birthweight score could also be treated as a z score drawn from a normal distribution. But, as we (Carr-Hill and Pritchard, 1983) have already argued, using data from this Aberdeen sample, the assumption of normal distributions of birthweight in gestation/sex/parity cells is a dangerous one on which to base clinical standards since, although the departures from normality are not very large, they effectively blur diagnostic criteria when the standards are used to assess individual babies (see chapter 9).

The issue is much less serious in the derivation and use of research standards. For, whilst the use of parametric methods such as analysis of variance used in these chapters in principle depends upon normal distributions of the error terms, the estimation of coefficients will be robust unless there are extreme departures from normality because of the large numbers involved.

A rather different kind of question is whether the statistically convenient assumption that the standardised score is drawn from a normal distribution, when it is known not to be the case (see table 9.3 in chapter 9), significantly affects the description of the population. This can be tested by examining the association between birthweight and its standardised birthweight score in each of the gestation/sex/parity cells. Unsurprisingly, the correlation coefficients in each of these cells are 1.00 as the standardised birthweight scores are a one-to-one mapping of birthweights. It is more interesting to examine the slope of the regression line: for one unit of the standardised birthweight score should be equivalent to one standard deviation of birthweight so that discrepancies between the estimated slope of the regression line and the standard deviation of birthweight for each cell reflect the effects of divergence from normality. The maximum difference observed at one standard deviation is 13.3 g for boys para 0 at 33 weeks (see figure 8.1). This is very small and confirms that, for the purpose of statistical manipulation, the data can be treated as normally distributed.

Having ensured that the assumption of normality provides a good fit for the data, it is then crucial to ensure that the correlation between the standardised birthweight scores and the factors controlled for (gestation, sex and parity 0; 1+) has disappeared. In these data there is *no* zero order correlation between the raw birthweight scores and the standardised birthweight scores; in contrast, the correlation between the standardised birthweight scores and birthweight controlling for gestation, sex and parity is nearly one (see table 8.2). It is also

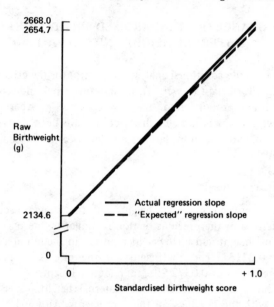

Figure 8.1　Raw birthweight against standardised birthweight score, boys, parity 0, 33 weeks' gestation

Table 8.2　Correlations between standardised birthweight scores and birthweight controlling for gestation, sex and parity (0/1+)

	Birthweight	Gestation	Sex	Parity
Zero order	0.871	0.0013	0.0007	−0.0003
	Controlling for	Gestation	Sex	Parity
1st order	NA	0.965	0.879	0.878
2nd order	Gestation	NA	0.977	0.975
Controlling	Sex	0.977	NA	0.886
for	Parity	0.975	0.886	NA
3rd order	0.988	NA	NA	NA

of interest to examine whether there is a correlation between parity – taking all its possible values – and the standards: the observed coefficient at 0.0096 is not significant. This would suggest that multiparity does not have an effect over and above the difference from primiparae (see also later in this chapter).

These standardised birthweight scores do, therefore, effectively 'take out' the effects of gestation, sex and parity (0/1+) from the birthweight distributions and also have the convenient property of having a mean 0 and a standard deviation of 1. The next question is whether or not the other 'intermediate' factors and, in particular, maternal height and weight-for-height, have an effect over and above these three factors.

THE COVARIANCE OF STANDARDISED BIRTHWEIGHT SCORES, MATERNAL HEIGHT AND z WEIGHT

This section reports the additional analyses to control for the effects of maternal height and weight-for-height (z weight). Because maternal mid-term weights are only available for a proportion of the data collected at Aberdeen, the standardised birthweight scores used in this section have been derived in the way discussed in the previous section, but are restricted to the subsample for whom weights are available.

The effect of maternal height

The correlation between maternal height and the standardised birthweight scores (SBS) derived in the previous section is similar to the partial correlation between maternal height and birthweight reported in the initial analysis (r_{bwt} = 0.2282; r_{SBS} = 0.2215). The coefficient for the effects of maternal height represents an increment of 0.0372 SBS/cm maternal height.

Table 8.3 shows the coefficients for maternal height for each gestational week, together with the F values for the coefficients. Although the coefficients are by no means identical, differences from the overall coefficient are only

Table 8.3   Coefficients for the effects of height on SBS by
individual weeks of gestation with F values for the
estimates and residual sums of squares

Week of gestation	Coefficient	F	SS resid.	N
32	0.0155	0.20	33.79	34
33	0.0156	0.51	62.36	62
34	0.0432	9.18†	90.00	99
35	0.0114	0.61	158.53	159
36	0.0473	27.43*	295.62	318
37	0.0311	27.35*	666.99	687
38	0.0347	94.11*	1698.71	1791
39	0.0366	230.92*	998.66	4231
40	0.0396	378.27*	5535.59	5916
41	0.0394	222.46*	3354.26	3749
42	0.0394	24.64*	460.82	482
All weeks 0.0372		1002.37	16 566.52	17528

*$P < 0.001$.
†$P < 0.025$.

substantial at the early gestational ages and these coefficients are not significant. This relatively uniform pattern suggests that it might be appropriate to use a single coefficient to control for the effects of height over the whole range of gestational ages. A Chow test of the comparison between the separate effects of maternal height within regression models for each gestational week, as against a single coefficient over the whole range of gestational ages, is non-significant ($F_{10,17515} = 1.205$, $0.20 > p > 0.10$). For statistical purposes it is, therefore, appropriate to use a single coefficient to control for the effects of height.

The effect of maternal z weight

The correlation between maternal z weight and standardised birthweight score is also similar to the correlation between maternal z weight and birthweight ($r_{bwt} = 0.2232$; $r_{SBS} = 0.2340$). The coefficient for the effects of maternal z weight is 0.2444, an increment of 0.2444 standardised birthweight scores for each standard deviation in weight-for-height.

In contrast to the effects of maternal height, however, the effects of maternal z weight are not uniform for each gestational week (table 8.4). For babies born

Table 8.4   Coefficients for the effects of z-weight on SBS by individual weeks of gestation with F values for the estimates

Week of gestation	Coefficient	F	SS$_{resid.}$	N
32	−0.0728	0.05	12.95	13
33	−0.0266	0.01	21.99	22
34	−0.0254	0.02	26.83	27
35	0.1409	1.23	52.19	54
36	0.1104	1.61	109.01	111
37	0.2566	18.26*	206.98	229
38	0.3387	64.57*	504.89	563
39	0.2581	95.76*	1115.66	1203
40	0.2684	111.56*	1525.45	1630
41	0.1812	70.19*	984.06	1013
42	0.2052	5.29†	129.83	135
All weeks	0.2444	17.49*	4707.47	4995

*$P < 0.001$.
†$P < 0.025$.

before the 37th week of gestation, the effects are markedly smaller than for those born at 37 weeks or later. Moreover, none of the 't' values for the coefficients between 32 and 36 weeks gestation are significant. A Chow test comparing the separate effects of maternal weight within regression models for each gestational week confirms that it is not appropriate to treat the effect of maternal z weight as uniform over all gestational weeks ($F_{10,4992} = 1.872, p < 0.05$)

The pattern of effects would seem to suggest that the effects of maternal weight are concentrated among 'term' babies and, indeed, a Chow test comparing two separate equations for pre-term babies (without a maternal weight variable) and for term babies, confirms that this split is appropriate ($F_{1,4992} = p >$ 0.10). However, it is not obvious that a uniform coefficient for maternal weight among term gestational weeks is appropriate; thus the coefficients of maternal z weight upon standardised birthweight scores for 38 and 41 weeks are significantly different from the overall coefficient of 0.2532 for all 'term' babies. However, a Chow test comparing the separate effects of maternal weight within regression models for each of the term gestational weeks confirms that it is statistically appropriate to treat the effect of maternal z weight as uniform over the term gestational weeks ($F_{5,\infty} = 1.63, p > 0.10$).

Interaction between maternal height and z weight

The significant variation in the coefficients for the individual gestational weeks, however, prompted us to explore further. Although maternal height and z weight are not significantly correlated, the interaction term for the effects of maternal height and z weight upon the standardised birthweight scores among term babies is significant ($F = 7.13, p < 0.01$). A Chow test comparing models with and without an interaction term confirms that it is appropriate to include the interaction of height and z weight ($F_{1,\infty} = 6.40, p < 0.001$) but the inclusion of interaction terms for the separate gestational weeks does not lead to any significant improvement ($F_{5,\infty} = 1.88, p > 0.10$).

Table 8.5 shows the coefficients for maternal height, maternal z weight and the interaction term derived from the model incorporating the interaction. The massively increased coefficient for maternal z weight is offset by the negative interaction term. Table 8.5 also shows the coefficients for maternal z weight by gestation. The significant differences in the coefficients for separate gestational weeks are no longer apparent.

The effects of the interaction term can be understood by comparing the estimates for maternal height by maternal z weight categories derived from models with and without the interaction term. Table 8.6 reports the discrepancies – that is, the estimate with interaction minus the estimate without interaction – in maternal height by z weight categories for this Aberdeen sample. The missing cells are those for which no observations were available. The effect of the interaction is such that the estimates based on a simple additive model are reduced for women who are short and light for their height and for women who are tall and heavy for their height; whilst they are increased for women who are tall and light for their height and for women who are short and heavy for their height. Table 8.7 shows the estimated standardised birthweight scores for maternal height/z weight cells derived from the model including the interaction term for the Aberdeen sample. The estimates show the substantial effects of maternal height and z weight. For example, the difference between a baby born to a woman of under 144 cm who is 1.5 standard deviations below the mean weight-for-height and a woman of over 175 cm who is 1.5 standard deviations above the mean weight-for-height is 1.98 SBS: if the mother were primiparous, giving

Table 8.5   Coefficients for maternal height, maternal z weight, and
their interaction (height × z weight) for babies born
later than 36 weeks' gestation ($N = 4768$)

	Coefficient	't'	SS
Model 1: Constant Effects Across Gestation			
Height	0.0356	16.25*	239.14
z weight	1.2094	3.37*	290.83
Height × z weight	−0.0060	−2.67†	6.34
Within and residual			4233.74
Model 2: Varying Slopes Within Gestational Ages			
Height	0.0356	16.26*	239.14
z weight			
37 weeks	1.2303	3.35*	
38 weeks	1.3058	3.62*	
39 weeks	1.2187	3.38*	
40 weeks	1.2377	3.44*	299.14
41 weeks	1.1588	3.20‡	
42 weeks	1.1951	3.24‡	
Height × z weight	−0.0061	3.24‡	6.47
Within and residual			4225.30

*$P < 0.001$.
†$P < 0.01$.
‡$P < 0.002$.

birth to a boy at 40 weeks gestation, this would be equivalent to an 'expected' difference in 'normal' birthweights of 855 g. Overall, the model suggests that the increment in standardised birthweight scores associated with increasing maternal height is decreased with increasing maternal z weight, and the increment associated with increasing maternal z weight is decreased with increasing maternal height.

The effects of maternal height and weight-for-height may be further gauged from table 8.8 which shows the estimated SBS for maternal height/mid-term weight cells derived from the model for the Aberdeen population. Over the range of maternal mid-term weights between 55 kg and 79.9 kg, the increment associated with increasing maternal mid-term weight is 0.84 SBS for women less than 144 cm and 0.23 SBS for women over 175 cm. Complementarily, over the range of maternal heights, the increment associated with increasing maternal height is 1.00 SBS for women weighing between 55 kg and 59.9 kg, and 0.39 SBS for women weighing between 75 kg and 79.9 kg. For heavier women, the increment associated with increasing height over the whole range is never more than 0.13 SBS and the 'expected' standardised birthweight score for women of medium height (between 155 and 164 cm) are less than those for shorter women.

Table 8.6 Discrepancies between cell estimates of SBS in maternal height/z weight cells derived for the Aberdeen population from models (a) incorporating the interactive effects of height and z weight and (b) without the interaction term. (Discrepancy = a − b)

Height	z weight to −1.75	to −1.25	to −0.75	to −0.25	to +0.25	to +0.75	to +1.25	to +1.75	to +2.25	2.26 and above
to 144 cm	*	−0.14	−0.10	−0.05	0.00	+0.07	+0.11	+0.33	+0.21	*
to 149 cm	−0.11	−0.09	−0.07	−0.04	0.00	+0.03	+0.06	+0.23	+0.15	+0.20
to 154 cm	−0.11	−0.06	−0.04	−0.02	0.00	+0.03	+0.04	+0.18	+0.09	+0.13
to 159 cm	−0.04	−0.02	−0.02	−0.01	0.00	+0.01	+0.01	+0.02	+0.03	+0.05
to 164 cm	+0.03	+0.02	+0.01	+0.01	0.00	−0.01	−0.02	−0.04	−0.02	−0.03
to 169 cm	+0.08	+0.07	+0.04	+0.02	0.00	−0.02	−0.04	−0.06	−0.09	−0.10
to 174 cm	*	+0.10	+0.07	+0.03	0.00	−0.03	−0.07	−0.10	−0.07	−0.22
175 cm and above	*	*	+0.10	+0.05	−0.01	−0.07	−0.11	−0.14	*	−0.37

* = insufficient observations.

Table 8.7 Estimates of SBS in height/z weight cells derived from the model for the effects of height and z weight (including height × weight interaction) for the Aberdeen population

Height	z weight									
	to −1.75	to −1.25	to −0.75	to −0.25	to +0.25	to +0.75	to +1.25	to +1.75	to +2.25	2.26 and above
to 144 cm	*	−1.13	−1.01	−0.74	−0.66	−0.44	−0.27	−0.05	+0.20	−*
to 149 cm	−0.95	−0.90	−0.75	−0.58	−0.42	−0.27	−0.13	+0.04	+0.26	+0.54
to 154 cm	−0.96	−0.68	−0.54	−0.40	−0.26	−0.11	+0.03	+0.18	+0.31	+0.62
to 159 cm	−0.64	−0.46	−0.35	−0.22	−0.10	+0.03	+0.17	+0.31	+0.43	+0.76
to 164 cm	−0.53	−0.24	−0.14	−0.05	+0.07	+0.19	+0.32	+0.44	+0.54	+0.76
to 169 cm	−0.13	−0.02	+0.04	+0.14	+0.24	+0.35	+0.45	+0.54	+0.67	+0.83
to 174 cm	*	+0.19	+0.26	+0.32	+0.40	+0.51	+0.60	+0.70	+0.75	+0.98
175 cm and above	*	*	+0.45	+0.52	+0.64	+0.70	+0.78	+0.86	*	+1.13

* = insufficient observations.

Table 8.8 Estimates of SBS in height/weight cells derived from model of the effects of height and z weight (including height × z weight interaction)

Height	Weight (kg) to 34.9	to 39.9	to 44.9	to 49.9	to 54.9	to 59.9	to 64.9	to 69.9	to 74.9	to 79.9	to 84.9	to 89.9	90.0 and above
to 144 cm	*	−*	−1.06	−0.91	−0.68	−0.64	−0.32	−0.15	−0.01	+0.20	*	*	*
to 149 cm	*	−1.05	−0.85	−0.71	−0.52	−0.35	−0.17	+0.02	+0.23	+0.31	+0.64	*	+0.82
to 154 cm	−2.02	*	−0.77	−0.61	−0.44	−0.28	−0.11	+0.05	+0.24	+0.41	+0.58	+0.80	+1.01
to 159 cm	−*	*	−0.63	−0.47	−0.33	−0.19	−0.05	+0.09	+0.24	+0.38	+0.51	+0.64	+1.07
to 164 cm	−1.18	*	−0.40	−0.32	−0.21	−0.09	+0.03	+0.14	+0.25	+0.38	+0.49	+0.61	+0.81
to 169 cm	−*	*	*	−0.13	−0.06	+0.03	+0.14	+0.24	+0.34	+0.44	+0.54	+0.66	+0.81
to 174 cm	*	*	*	*	+0.19	+0.19	+0.27	+0.34	+0.42	+0.52	+0.61	+0.70	+0.91
175 cm and above	*	*	*	*	*	+0.36	+0.46	+0.52	+0.64	+0.59	+0.75	+0.84	+0.95

* = insufficient observations.

The appropriate statistical test for comparing and contrasting any of these estimates, which are derived from a combination of parameters of a multivariate statistical model, is not obvious. However, the differences in the increments, when translated into grams of baby, are clearly substantial and different from each other and from a notional overall value.

Given that we had originally advocated an essentially descriptive analytic strategy, it is incumbent upon us to verify that the pattern of effects due to maternal height and z weight, as represented by these estimates from a statistical model does, in fact, reflect the observed variations in birthweight with maternal size. Table 8.9 illustrates this comparison between estimated and actual

Table 8.9   Observed and estimated mean SBS for women weighing between 75 and 79.9 kg by height

Height	Estimated SBS	Observed SBS	N
to 154 cm	0.41	0.49	18
to 159 cm	0.38	0.31	53
to 164 cm	0.38	0.36	83
to 169 cm	0.44	0.46	60

mean standardised birthweight scores for women between 75 kg and 79.9 kg (for those maternal height cells where there are sufficient numbers); this weight group has been chosen as being of particular interest because of the apparently anomalous reversal in the pattern of effects over the range of maternal heights. In fact, the pattern predicted by the estimates (including the interaction term) of a decrease in standardised birthweight score with increased maternal height followed by an increase in standardised birthweight score as maternal height increases even further, corresponds well with the pattern observed in the data. The closeness of the fit, both in terms of the values and more especially in terms of the pattern of effects, is replicated for other maternal height groups and maternal z weight groups, whenever there are sufficient numbers in the cells.

THE EFFECTS OF HIGHER PARITIES AND MATERNAL AGE

The issue for this section is whether or not any of the two remaining factors classified as 'intermediate' in chapter 5 affect standardised birthweight scores after controlling for gestation, sex and parity (0 : 1+) in the manner described above. These are the variations among multiparae and maternal age.

The effect of higher parity amongst multiparae

The argument and analysis have, so far, been conducted in terms of the dichotomy (0 : 1+). Earlier, in chapter 3, attention was drawn to the inconclusive discussion in the literature: the treatment until now has relied upon a particular view as to the role of parity and the simple observation that higher parous women tend to be heavier. Various checks along the way confirmed that parity (taking all its possible values) does not have a significant effect if entered into the general model *after* both maternal height and z weight. Nevertheless, that particular ordering is, more or less, arbitrary.

The issue is best explored among multiparae. Table 8.10 shows the pattern of standardised birthweight scores with parity; and indeed, they do appear to increase from parity 1 to higher parities when the standardisation procedure

Table 8.10   Mean standardised birthweight scores by parity (0, 1, 2, 3+)

Parity	Mean	SD	N
0	−0.001	0.999	7705
1	−0.024	0.983	6695
2	0.048	1.02	2338
3+	0.048	1.07	790
All	−0.001	1.00	17528

(that is, standardisation as between parities 0 and 1+) should have controlled for this effect. At the same time, mean maternal weight and z weight increases substantially from parity 1 to higher parities which might account for this anomalous observation. This is confirmed by analysis using the multivariate model. Parity $(1, 2, \ldots, 9)$ has a significant effect upon standardised birthweight scores if entered first in the model ($F = 2.35, p = 0.012$) or after maternal height and before maternal z weight ($F = 1.85$, $p = 0.05$). However, among multiparae for whom there is maternal weight data ($N = 2452$), parity no longer has a significant effect if entered in the model after *both* maternal height and z weight ($F = 1.32, p = 0.16$).

It is not, *prima facie*, obvious which version to adopt or believe. In principle, the theoretical argument in chapter 5 would ascribe precedence in analysing birthweight distributions to variations in parity over variations in maternal z weight and, therefore, to the former version. It is, however, possible that women who continue to higher parities after parity 1 have heavier babies throughout their reproductive career than those who have a shorter reproductive career independently of increases in maternal weight and z weight (see Billewicz and Thomson, 1973).

There is (some) supporting evidence from a career-wise study conducted by one of the authors, also based on the Aberdeen Maternity and Neonatal Data

Bank, of women whose first recorded pregnancy was between 1958 and 1977. Carr-Hill and Samphier (1983) studied 13 222 women who had had a sequence of uninterrupted singleton live births of certain gestation following their first pregnancy of whom 5011 had two, 1196 had three, and 265 had four or more live births. They standardised the birthweights for gestational age, maternal height, sex of infant and whether first or later born on the basis of the Altman–Coles version of the fetal growth standards developed by Thomson *et al.* (1968). The relevant results (taken from their table 7) are presented as table 8.11. Note

Table 8.11   Means and standard deviations of standardised birthweight scores and maternal height according to number of live births

	No. of Live Births							
	2		3		4		All	
	Mean	SD	Mean	SD	Mean	SD	Mean	SD
1st birth	100.63	9.74	101.30	9.85	100.83	9.65	100.76	9.75
2nd birth	100.13	9.32	100.58	9.06	100.87	8.83	100.26	9.21
3rd birth			100.70	9.66	101.23	9.20	100.80	9.45
4th birth					101.21	9.31	101.21	9.31
Maternal height	158.55	9.75	158.05	10.88	156.76	16.11	158.01	11.23

that Altman–Coles birthweight scores have a mean of 100 and a standard deviation of 10 (henceforth, an AC standard deviation).

It can be seen that the first and second births of those who had three or four or more births was slightly heavier than those who had just two births; similarly, the third birth of those who had four or more births was also slightly heavier than those who had only three births. At the same time, within each of the equiparous groups there is no obvious trend within multiparae: thus, whilst there is an *increase* of 0.012 and 0.036 of an AC standard deviation between the second and third births of three sibships and four sibships, there is a *decrease* of 0.002 of an AC standard deviation (that is, about 9 grams between the third and fourth births of four sibships).

But the relative numbers of those with two, three and four births are such that, if *all sibships are combined* – as they are in a cross-sectional study such as ours – there is a trend from parity to parity among multiparae. The average standardised birthweight scores among the 6472 women who had two or more live births are 100.76 at first birth, 100.26 at second birth, 100.80 at third birth, and 101.21 at fourth birth: among multiparae, there is, therefore an increase of 10% of an AC standard deviation between the second and fourth births (that is, about 22 grams *per parity*). This just happens to correspond to the effect noted in table 8.10 above.

The effect of maternal age

The review of literature in chapter 3 reported conflicting conclusions about the effects of maternal age on birthweight, mostly related to differences between populations.

Table 8.12 shows the coefficients for maternal age in gestation/sex/parity groups after adjusting for the effects of maternal height and z weight, together with their standard errors, 't' values and the significance of the 't' tests. The 't' values are only once significant (for boys, parity 1+, born at 34 weeks gestation). The conclusion is that the incorporation of maternal age will not significantly affect the estimates incorporating gestation, sex, parity and maternal height and z weight and so can be discarded in future analysis. It is important to note that this is not the same as saying that maternal age has no effect on birthweight in this population; it is only a statement that it does not affect the relationship between the statistical model and the observations that the model describes.

STANDARDS INCORPORATING MATERNAL HEIGHT AND z WEIGHT ('CORRECTED STANDARDISED BIRTHWEIGHT SCORES')

At the end of the previous chapter, the attempt to find a simple functional form relating birthweight to gestation was abandoned in the face of irreducible anomalies at 32, 37 and 42 weeks. Instead, it was argued that it was preferable to standardise directly in terms of the empirically observed distribution in gestation/sex/parity cells. In principle, the same argument applies here: if one wants to adjust the standards for the effects of maternal height and z weight then this should be done directly in terms of the empirically observed distributions of standardised birthweight scores in maternal height by maternal z weight cells.

However, maternal height and z weight are continuous variables and such standards would be sensitive to the categorisation employed. More importantly, the numbers in maternal height by maternal z weight cells, in the Aberdeen sample at least, quickly become very small as maternal height and z weight diverge from their mean values. For these reasons, a less desirable technique — using the values derived from the model of the effects of maternal height and z weight — has been used to control for the effects of maternal height and z weight in the studies reported later in this monograph which require this adjustment (see chapters 10 and 11).

This model-fitting procedure is *bound* to introduce some error but the particular fit has not given rise to any systematic irreducible anomalies at particular gestational weeks or at certain points of the maternal height/z weight distribution. It is true that the statistical tests showed that the assumption of a uniform coefficient over all gestational ages was appropriate only for maternal height and not for maternal z weight (even when restricted to babies delivered

Table 8.12 Coefficients for the regression of 'corrected' (for maternal size) standardised birthweight scores on maternal age in gestation/sex/parity cells

Weeks gest.	Boys, para 0			Girls, para 0			Boys, para 1+			Girls, para 1+		
	Coeff.	t	p	Coeff.	t	p	Coeff.	t	p	Coeff.	t	p
32	-0.0006	-0.04	NS	-0.0016	-0.06	NS	*	*	*	-0.0043	-0.22	NS
33	0.0002	0.02	NS	0.0020	0.13	NS	0.0075	0.54	NS	0.0024	0.17	NS
34	0.0034	0.27	NS	-0.0142	-0.86	NS	0.0045	0.33	NS	-0.0172	-1.02	NS
35	-0.0044	-0.37	NS	-0.0023	-0.22	NS	-0.0023	-0.20	NS	0.0027	0.25	NS
36	-0.0009	-0.11	NS	-0.0072	-0.88	NS	-0.0029	-0.29	NS	0.0040	0.43	NS
37	-0.0009	-0.12	NS	-0.0039	-0.50	NS	0.0016	0.21	NS	0.0020	0.26	NS
38	-0.0026	-0.41	NS	-0.0059	-0.86	NS	0.0000	0.00	NS	0.0017	0.26	NS
39	-0.0026	-0.42	NS	-0.0032	-0.50	NS	-0.0015	-0.24	NS	0.0008	0.12	NS
40	-0.0010	-0.17	NS	-0.0044	-0.69	NS	-0.0012	-0.20	NS	0.0000	0.00	NS
41	-0.0034	-0.53	NS	-0.0038	-0.55	NS	-0.0025	-0.39	NS	0.0002	0.03	NS
42	-0.0032	-0.32	NS	-0.0047	-0.52	NS	0.0007	0.08	NS	-0.0037	-0.40	NS

at term). But the apparently anomalous variations in standardised birthweight scores when both maternal height and z weight are considered can best be understood by the incorporation of an interaction term among babies alongside a *uniform* coefficient for maternal z weight amongst term babies.

For any individual birthweight, the 'standard' has, as it were, two components. The standardised birthweight score locates the birthweight in the distribution of birthweights in a particular gestation/sex/parity cell of the population. The maternal height and z weight adjustment gives an expected value of the standardised birthweight score for a woman of a particular height and weight-for-height. Where the expected value derived from the model for the effects of maternal height and z weight and the actual standardised birthweight score are the same, the corrected standardised birthweight for that baby should equal 0.

Thus, for each individual the corrected standard equals the standardised birthweight score less the expected value derived from the analysis of the effects of maternal height and z weight. Table 8.13 shows the 'correction' procedure

Table 8.13   Examples of the calculation of the maternal size correction for individual cases for boy, first-born babies of 40 weeks' gestation (cell mean birthweight 3420.5 g standard deviation 414.4)

	Woman 1	Woman 2
Maternal Size — height	152.5 cm	80.5 kg
— weight	47.5 kg	176.0 cm
Birthweight	3167.7 g	3500 g
Raw standardised birthweight score	$\dfrac{3167.7 - 3420.5}{414.4}$ $= -0.61$	$\dfrac{3500 - 3420.5}{414.4}$ $= +0.19$
Correction factor from table 8.8	-0.61	$+0.75$
Corrected standardised birthweight score	$-0.61 - (-0.61)$ $= 0.0$	$0.19 - (+0.75)$ $= -0.56$

for two examples. Another method of making the correction for maternal size is shown in chapter 9. Standards calculated in this way ought effectively to control for the effects of gestation, sex, parity, maternal height and maternal z weight: these variables ought not to be significantly correlated with the standards and, such correlations as there are, are not significant.

The development of the maternal height/z weight adjustment was on the basis of standardised birthweight scores rather than raw birthweights, and it is also important to check that there are no anomalies arising from this procedure. Because of the nature of maternal height and z weight, the adjustment is statistical rather than 'empirical', and it is possible to check that this is at least the equivalent of statistically controlling for the effects of maternal height and z weight on raw birthweight. This can be done for a particular gestation/sex/parity group by specifying a multiple regression in which the effects of maternal height and z weight and their interaction on birthweight are entered first followed by the standardised birthweight scores. Ideally, the correlation coefficient in such a model should be 1.0 and the slope of the regression of standardised birthweight score on birthweight ought to equal the standard deviation of birthweight in that gestation/sex/parity cell. By way of illustration, the results of such an analysis for babies born at 40 weeks gestation are presented in table 8.14. They are

Table 8.14   Correlation coefficient (multiple R) for the regression of height z weight, the interaction height × z weight, and standards on birthweight; the coefficient for standards and the standard deviation of birthweight, babies at 40 weeks' gestation

	Multiple R	Coefficient standards	Standard deviation birthweight
Boys parity 0	0.9989	425.77	424.72
Girls parity 0	0.9992	389.40	390.71
Boys parity 1+	0.9991	443.06	444.64
Girls parity 1+	0.9989	397.18	397.64

typical of the results for the other gestational weeks and confirm that standards incorporating the maternal height/z weight adjustment are equivalent to the statistical control of the effects of maternal height and z weight on birthweight. They further lend some evidence about the relationship between the standards derived in this way and the values for birthweight they are intended to describe.

EMPIRICAL BIRTHWEIGHT STANDARDS FOR RESEARCH PURPOSES – A SUMMARY

The intention of this and the previous chapter has been to argue for a particular approach to the development of birthweight standards and to illustrate that approach from the material from the Aberdeen population. The development of these standards has attempted to take seriously the conclusion that birthweight standards ought to represent a description of the distribution of birthweights in a particular population. This is in contrast to an appeal to the universality of the effects of factors related to birthweight because of a postulated fetal growth process, or to the universal appropriateness of models derived from statistical theory.

For the purposes of this illustration, however, the analysis in the latter half of this chapter has involved something of a compromise. The statistical adjustment for the effects of maternal height and z weight is the consequence of the nature of the variables and the limits of the sample. Each compromise, however, has been referred back to the raw data of the sample and its effects carefully checked in an attempt to ensure that serious bias is not introduced by the procedure adopted.

For purposes where the maternal height/weight adjustment is not required, for example, where the research interest is with factors related to maternal size, the 'standards' used would simply be the standardised birthweight scores for gestation/sex/parity groups calculated as the 'observed birthweight minus cell mean' divided by the standard deviation of the cell (for the general formula, see chapter 6, page 69). In some cases, the added assumption that their distribution is normal may not materially affect the descriptive power of the standards, and in this case the use of the equivalent normal distribution would be more convenient.

The illustrative standards developed in these chapters have been developed for parity defined as 0; 1+. Whilst in this population the effects of parities within the '1+' category are still apparent, these effects are explicable either in terms of maternal size or because higher parities select for more efficient reproducers (as distinct from higher pregnancy number which might incorporate a succession of wasted pregnancies). Thus, care should be taken in cross-sectional studies when the standards are used without an adjustment for maternal size since the effect which is the subject of research may be confounded by an apparent effect of multiparity. In clinical use, although this 'effect' of higher multiparity is not large, it may represent a problem in the assessment of babies of highly parous women when maternal weight data was not collected at the appropriate time. In these cases, the assessment should be informed by an inspection of the mother's previous obstetric history.

The maternal height/weight adjustment itself has been derived from a statistical model which assessed the effects of maternal height and weight in terms of standardised birthweight scores and, as noted, represents a compromise in the overall empirical approach. The adjustment was separately calculated for pre-term and for term babies. In the case of term babies, the effects of both maternal height and weight-for-height form part of the adjustment. For babies born before 37 weeks, however, the effects of maternal weight-for-height were not found to be significant in the Aberdeen population, and the adjustment for maternal size is only an adjustment for maternal height. It was further noted that, because of the interaction between the effects of maternal height and z weight, the use of the coefficients of either to assess their independent effects would be inappropriate.

Overall, we believe that standardised birthweight scores developed along the lines of this and the previous chapter represent a significant departure from current practice and have much to offer the researcher (for further discussion, see chapter 12). We also believe that the clinician will profit from a recasting of birthweight standards in this form. The particular issues involved in their practical exploitation by the clinician are the subject of the next chapter.

SECTION 4

The use of birthweight standards

The three chapters in this section discuss and illustrate the use of the birthweight standards derived in the previous section. Chapter 9 shows how such standards form the basis of clinical standards and discusses the difficulties inherent in their application. Chapters 10 and 11 are intended as illustrative studies of the research use of standards.

9
Clinical standards for birthweight

INTRODUCTION

The preceding chapters have shown how much of the variation in birthweight can be accounted for by the 'normal' factors of gestation and sex and the 'intermediate' factors of parity, maternal height and maternal weight-for-height. The intention of this chapter is to illustrate how such standardised birthweight scores could be used to derive clinical standards (corrected for maternal height and maternal weight-for-height) and to compare these standards with the empirical distributions of birthweight. A comprehensive set of local clinical standards have been derived for the Aberdeen District population, using the method described.

The use of standardised birthweight for the assessment of individual babies has been noted in chapter 1. The information provided by the standardised birthweight represents an 'expected' value for birthweight and a quantitative assessment of any departure from the expected value. The *clinical* significance of such departures is a matter for clinical judgement and empirical research. Thomson and Billewicz (1976) have raised doubts about the value of the concept of 'lightness-for-dates' in paediatric assessment, particularly in the assessment of the risk of perinatal death (see also Hellier and Goldstein, 1979) but conclude that knowledge of birthweight for gestation gives useful clinical guidance to neonatal paediatricians (p. 74) as part of an overall assessment of the baby's intrauterine development.

CLINICAL STANDARDS ASSUMING THE NORMAL DISTRIBUTION OF BIRTHWEIGHT IN GESTATION/SEX/PARITY CELLS

The standards developed here reflect the convention of identifying the birthweights corresponding to the 5th, 10th, 90th and 95th percentiles of the cumulative distribution of birthweights in particular gestation/sex/parity cells. The classic method of doing this is to assume that birthweight within any gestation/sex/parity cells follows a normal distribution so that the location of any particu-

123

Table 9.1 Means, standard deviation and normal equivalent 5th, 10th, 90th and 95th percentiles of birthweight in sex parity and gestation cells

Standard with only height known ($N = 17\,528$)

Weeks of gestation and parity	Boys							Girls						
	Mean	Standard deviation	N	Actual percentile				Mean	Standard deviation	N	Actual percentile			
				5th	10th	90th	95th				5th	10th	90th	95th
Para 0														
32	1843.1	321.8	13	1313.6	1429.7	2256.5	2372.6	1790.0	496.2	8	973.5	1152.6	2427.4	2606.5
33	2134.6	340.1	13	1574.9	1697.7	2571.5	2694.2	1976.5	461.5	17	1217.1	1383.7	2569.3	2735.9
34	2360.3	502.1	32	1534.0	1923.9	2796.0	3185.9	2133.8	369.5	21	1525.8	1659.2	2609.4	2741.8
35	2489.8	440.2	44	1765.5	1924.4	3055.2	3214.1	2314.1	443.9	34	1583.7	1743.9	2884.3	3044.5
36	2701.2	431.2	77	1991.7	2147.3	3255.1	3410.7	2657.3	384.4	82	2024.8	2163.5	3151.1	3289.8
37	2927.9	435.9	169	2210.6	2367.9	3487.8	3645.2	2731.0	434.7	143	2015.7	2172.6	3289.4	3446.3
38	3177.5	402.5	392	2515.2	2660.5	3694.5	3839.8	3021.8	412.9	346	2342.4	2491.4	3552.2	3701.2
39	3302.6	428.8	901	2597.0	2751.8	3853.4	4008.2	3165.1	420.8	832	2472.7	2624.6	3705.6	3857.5
40	3420.5	414.4	1345	2738.6	2888.2	3952.8	4102.4	3287.9	399.8	1286	2630.0	2774.4	3801.4	3945.8
41	3508.2	416.3	854	2823.2	2973.5	4042.9	4193.2	3379.6	393.6	864	2731.9	2874.0	3885.2	4027.3
42	3475.0	454.8	111	2726.6	2890.8	4059.2	4223.4	3340.5	398.4	121	2294.4	2436.5	3447.7	3589.8
Para 1+														
32	1970.0	351.3	5	1391.9	1518.8	2421.2	2548.1	1902.5	289.7	8	1425.8	1530.4	2274.6	2379.2
33	2126.9	339.9	16	1567.6	1690.3	2563.5	2686.2	1970.6	301.8	16	1473.9	1582.9	2358.3	2467.2
34	2382.9	277.6	28	1926.1	2026.3	2739.5	2839.7	2353.3	408.7	18	1680.8	1828.3	2878.3	3025.8
35	2590.0	382.7	46	1960.3	2098.4	3081.6	3219.7	2550.9	465.3	35	1785.2	1953.2	3148.6	3316.6
36	2843.5	440.8	84	2118.2	2277.3	3409.7	3568.8	2640.2	418.6	75	1951.4	2102.5	3177.9	3329.0
37	3045.8	500.8	200	2221.7	2402.5	3689.1	3869.9	2961.9	437.6	175	2241.8	2399.8	3523.9	3681.9
38	3308.8	420.6	562	2616.7	2768.5	3849.1	4000.9	3141.4	392.2	491	2489.0	2630.6	3638.2	3779.8
39	3397.8	435.1	1360	2681.8	2838.9	3956.7	4113.8	3292.6	419.9	1138	2601.7	2753.2	3831.9	3983.5
40	3546.3	424.8	1677	2847.3	3000.6	4091.9	4245.3	3406.6	422.8	1608	2710.9	2863.5	3949.7	4102.3
41	3647.4	436.6	1045	2928.9	3086.6	4208.2	4365.8	3484.3	431.7	986	2773.9	2929.8	4038.8	4194.7
42	3570.9	461.3	117	2811.3	2977.9	4162.9	4329.5	3469.1	437.4	133	2749.4	2907.3	4030.9	4188.8

lar percentile is completely determined (for example, the 5th percentile is given by $\bar{x} - 1.645$ SD$_x$, when $\bar{x}$ and SD$_x$ are the mean and standard deviation of the distribution in that particular cell. Table 9.1 gives, for each week of gestation within the four sex/parity groups, the means and standard deviations and the 5th, 10th, 90th and 95th percentiles calculated in this manner, for these data. To refer any birthweight to this distribution, the 'raw' birthweight should first be corrected for maternal height and maternal weight-for-height according to the coefficients estimated in the previous chapter and prescribed in table 8.8.

Two examples of this calculation are presented in table 9.2 (and cf. table 8.13). The first refers to an apparently light baby born to a smaller woman, the

Table 9.2

Para 0 boy 40 weeks (cell mean = 3420.5, standard deviation = 414.4)		
	Woman 1	Woman 2
Maternal size – height	152.5 cm	176.0 cm
– mid-term weight	47.5 kg	80.5 kg
Raw birthweight	3167.7 grams	3500 grams
Size correction from table 8.8	−0.61	+0.75
in grams of birthweight	−0.61 × 414.4 grams	+0.75 × 414.4 grams
	−252.8 grams	+310.8 grams
Corrected birthweight to be	3167.7 − (−252.8)	3500 − (+310.8)
referred to table 9.1	3420.5	3189.2
Corrected Standardised Birthweight Score	$\dfrac{3420.5 - 3420.5}{414.4}$	$\dfrac{3189.2 - 3420.5}{414.4}$
	= 0.0	= −0.56
Using table of z scores Centile	= 50th	29th

other to an apparently marginally heavy baby born to a larger woman (compare 3167.7 and 3500 grams to the cell mean of 3420.5 − see table 9.1). The corrections for maternal size are obtained by looking up the estimates in the appropriate row and column of table 8.8. Thus, the smaller mother would, on average, have a baby 0.61 of a standard deviation lighter and the larger mother would, on average, have a baby 0.75 of a standard deviation heavier than a mother of average height and weight. Given that the standard deviation for first born boys at 40 weeks gestation is 414.4 grams, the corrections to be subtracted from the raw birthweight are (−252.8) and (+310.8) grams for the smaller and heavier woman respectively. The corrected birthweights are therefore 3420.5 and 3189.2 for the smaller and heavier mother respectively. Finally, to obtain the standardised birthweight score, these corrected birthweights should be referred to the birthweight distribution in the cell by subtracting the cell mean of 3420.5 from the corrected birthweight and dividing the result by the standard deviation of 414.4. As can be seen the apparently lighter baby has a standardised birthweight score of 0.0 (i.e. is an exactly 'average' baby) and the apparently marginally heavy baby has a standardised birthweight of −0.56 (is a slightly light-for-dates baby).

If, further, one wants to locate the standardised birthweight distribution at a centile on the equivalent normal distribution, these values need to be referred to a table of z scores. The babies of the smaller and heavier mother are located at the 50th and 29th centile respectively. However, the clinical significance of the birthweights can be assessed more directly, by comparing the corrected birthweights with the 5th, 10th, 90th and 95th percentiles presented in table 9.1. In the case of these two examples, both mothers, in fact, have a baby in the bottom half of the distribution but above the 10th centile.

It is important to remember that this procedure introduces a slight distortion because of the assumption that the parameter estimates for maternal size are constant. Thus, whilst we have shown that these parameter estimates are statistically appropriate over the whole range of gestation, inspection of tables 8.3 and 8.4 does suggest that there might be some variation if coefficients estimated separately for each gestational week had been employed. This seems especially likely at the pre-term weeks, but remember that numbers are small. Any error introduced by the assumption here of constant coefficients would, of course, only ever be important at the extremes of the height/weight distribution in the pre-term weeks.

THE SIGNIFICANCE OF DEPARTURES FROM NORMALITY IN GESTATION/SEX/PARITY CELLS

The last step in the procedure described above involved referring the standardised birthweight score (whether corrected or not) to an assumed normal distribution for the purpose of deriving the familiar percentile equivalent to the raw birthweight. The validity of this procedure, of course, depends upon the extent to which the distributions can correctly be assumed to be normal within each gestation/sex/parity cell (see Carr-Hill and Pritchard, 1983). Note that this assumption of normality is not a serious issue for multivariate analysis (whether that of chapters 7 and 8 or in research studies such as those reported in chapters 10 and 11) which is concerned with the direction and size of effects for the *whole* of a sample and over the *complete* range of a distribution (for a more technical justification, see chapter 8, pages 102–103). But the clinician is concerned with *individual* cases and with the *extremes* of the distribution (for example, those cases falling below the 5th percentile). To make any assumption about the distributional form then becomes problematic.

Table 9.3 comments upon the usual assumption of normality by giving the values of skewness and kurtosis, together with the *p* values comparing these estimates to the corresponding normal distribution. It can be seen that the distribution of birthweight is significantly skewed in a quarter (11/44) of the

Table 9.3 Values of skewness and kurtosis for the distribution of birthweight in gestation/sex/parity cells

Standards with only height known ($N = 17\,528$)

Weeks of gestation and parity	Boys							Girls						
	Mean	Standard deviation	N	Skewness	p value	Kurtosis	p value	Mean	Standard deviation	N	Skewness	p value	Kurtosis	p value
Para 0														
32	1843.1	321.8	13	-0.2099	0.8283	-0.6653	0.5133	1790.0	496.2	8	0.5291	0.6036	-0.3956	0.6951
33	2134.6	340.1	13	-0.1507	0.8749	-0.4746	0.6407	1976.5	461.5	17	1.1173	0.2631	-0.2535	0.7957
34	2360.3	502.1	32	-1.4207	0.1518	-0.2231	0.8183	2133.8	369.5	21	-0.2677	0.7853	-0.0034	1.0000
35	2489.8	440.2	44	-1.0839	0.2782	-0.5758	0.5721	2314.1	443.9	34	1.2644	0.2035	3.0909	0.0025
36	2701.2	431.2	77	0.1128	0.9064	0.2015	0.8347	2657.3	384.4	82	0.5305	0.6026	-1.2959	0.1922
37	2927.9	435.9	169	0.8354	0.5914	0.7246	0.5241	2731.0	434.7	143	0.9271	0.6433	-0.7616	0.5470
38	3177.5	402.5	392	1.1711	0.2400	1.1830	0.2351	3021.8	412.9	346	-3.3159	0.0013	5.5778	0.0000
39	3302.6	428.8	901	2.2790	0.0215	2.5769	0.0099	3165.1	420.8	832	-1.7545	0.0758	9.9397	0.0000
40	3420.5	414.4	1345	-0.4475	0.6593	1.5611	0.1147	3287.9	399.8	1286	2.2061	0.0259	0.7490	0.5397
41	3508.2	416.3	854	3.5310	0.0008	1.2459	0.2104	3379.6	393.6	864	1.4907	0.1323	1.2130	0.2231
42	3475.0	454.8	111	1.9118	0.0530	2.3117	0.0198	3340.5	398.4	121	1.4134	0.1540	1.1258	0.2594
Para 1+														
32	1970.0	351.3	5	0.2391	0.8063	-0.4912	0.6293	1902.5	289.7	8	0.4041	0.6892	-0.3399	0.7339
33	2126.9	339.9	16	0.0416	0.9657	-0.7940	0.5668	1970.6	301.8	16	-0.6736	0.5079	-0.4767	0.6393
34	2382.9	277.6	28	-0.1151	0.9044	-0.2886	0.7702	2353.3	408.7	18	1.1477	0.2499	-0.1899	0.8437
35	2590.0	382.7	46	-0.6273	0.5379	2.8158	0.0052	2550.9	465.3	35	0.0354	0.9705	1.0950	0.2731
36	2843.5	440.8	84	-0.5412	0.5954	1.1891	0.2326	2640.2	418.6	75	-1.1135	0.2648	0.9214	0.6402
37	3045.8	500.8	200	-2.3394	0.0184	6.7201	0.0000	2961.9	437.6	175	2.0812	0.0353	1.6338	0.0985
38	3308.8	420.6	562	-0.0091	1.0000	5.3084	0.0000	3141.4	392.2	491	0.5561	0.5853	0.5464	0.5918
39	3397.8	435.1	1360	—	—	—	—	3292.6	419.9	1138	0.9068	0.6322	-0.0161	1.0000
40	3546.3	424.8	1677	3.1488	0.0021	3.8228	0.0003	3406.6	422.8	1608	2.0753	0.0358	1.3618	0.1700
41	3647.4	436.6	1045	1.3182	0.1845	1.1146	0.2643	3484.3	431.7	986	2.6789	0.0075	2.1163	0.0324
42	3570.9	461.3	117	-0.7107	0.5155	-0.3645	0.7166	3469.1	437.4	133	1.2760	0.1993	-0.0092	1.0000

cells and is significantly platykurtic in 12 of the cells. It is of particular importance to note that more than half the cells (14/24) for gestations of 37 weeks or
over show statistically significant departures from normality. While the value
for the significance of these departures reflects the larger numbers born in the
later weeks of gestation it also means that larger numbers of individual babies
would be inappropriately assessed under the assumption of normality.

To investigate this further, the empirically observed 5th, 10th, 90th and
95th percentiles within each week of gestation for the four sex/parity groups
are given in table 9.4. The differences between those empirical percentiles and
those derived from the normal distributions are given in table 9.5 and the actual
empirical percentages which fall into the estimated 5th, 10th, 90th and 95th
percentile are given in table 9.6. Whilst the differences given in table 9.5 do not
appear to be very large, the discrepancies in table 9.6 could be serious if the
percentiles derived from the normal distributions are used as part of the decision
making in clinical management. For example, the estimated normal equivalent
5th percentile for mothers of first born boys delivering at 41 weeks actually
includes 3.5% of the 854 first born males born at 41 weeks.

If the distributions of birthweight in this cell were normal, it would be
assumed that about 43 of the cases fall below a notional 5th percentile. In
fact, only 3.5% (i.e. 31 cases) of the observed birthweight are below 2884.1
grammes which is the normal equivalent 5th percentile. Hence, 12 cases, which
on the basis of the empirical distributions are below the 5th percentile of their
own gestation/sex/parity cell (which is the usual clinical diagnostic criterion of
'light-for-dates') would not be so classified if the birthweights in that cell were
assumed to be normally distributed. This result might be a peculiarity of this
data set: it seems doubtful (for further discussion, see Carr-Hill and Pritchard,
1983).

DISCUSSION

Of course, in actual clinical practice, the assessment of an individual baby will
take into account many factors besides the normal equivalent percentile to the
standardised birthweight score. Thus, the potential for the misallocation of
resources implied by these discrepancies is exaggerated by the comparisons
noted above. The whole problem can be avoided by using the standardised
birthweight score (whether corrected or not) itself, *without* translating to a
normal equivalent percentile. Nevertheless, the usual criteria for a diagnosis
of 'light-for-dates' do rely on normal equivalent percentiles, and the above
analysis shows that, in both a statistical and a substantial sense, the assumption
of normality is not appropriate.

It would be possible to use the observed distributions to provide diagnostic
criteria for the assessment of departures from the expected birthweight. Such
a course would entail considerable difficulties in an adjustment for maternal

Table 9.4 Empirically observed 5th, 10th, 90th and 95th percentiles of birthweight in gestation/sex/parity cells

Standards with only height known (N = 17 528)

Weeks of gestation and parity		Boys				Estimated percentile			Girls				Estimated percentile		
		Mean	Median	N	5th	10th	90th	95th	N	Median	Mean	5th	10th	90th	95th
Para 0	32	1843.1	1884.3	13	1309.7	1425.7	2237.3	2372.6	8	1720.4	1790.0	–	1125.9	2529.1	–
	33	2134.6	2192.9	13	1615.8	1636.3	2608.5	2731.0	17	1886.9	1976.5	1349.7	1439.2	2603.3	2886.8
	34	2360.3	2429.5	32	1421.3	1589.3	3011.0	3052.2	21	2144.1	2133.8	1434.3	1693.9	2609.7	2761.2
	35	2489.8	2518.8	44	1662.9	1978.4	3026.5	3113.6	34	2266.0	3314.1	1701.9	1815.6	2751.4	3015.1
	36	2701.2	2690.5	77	1930.1	2187.1	3300.9	3472.2	82	2664.9	2657.3	2007.8	2211.6	3192.2	3306.8
	37	2927.9	2893.1	169	2275.9	2362.8	3449.4	3666.8	143	2748.5	2731.0	2044.6	2261.2	3344.2	3517.4
	38	3177.5	3187.5	392	2494.1	2695.1	3686.6	3800.5	346	3032.1	3021.8	2362.2	2527.1	3516.5	3681.4
	39	3302.6	3285.4	901	2616.8	2788.3	3859.7	4073.9	832	3154.6	3165.1	2534.3	2660.4	3690.8	3880.1
	40	3420.5	3413.6	1345	2716.3	2882.0	3958.9	4103.9	1286	3277.9	3287.9	2648.5	2788.4	3787.6	3927.5
	41	3508.2	3480.5	854	2884.1	3008.9	4049.1	4257.2	864	3369.7	3379.6	2789.6	2907.6	3890.9	4048.3
	42	3475.0	3407.1	111	2773.2	2909.1	4074.9	4169.3	121	3324.6	3340.5	2665.9	2864.3	3856.3	4014.9
Para 1+	32	1970.0	1875.7	5	–	1530.1	2472.7	–	8	1830.2	1902.5	–	1544.0	2323.5	–
	33	2126.9	2126.9	16	1620.0	1669.4	2571.2	2697.4	16	2009.6	1970.6	1425.1	1515.6	2338.8	–
	34	2382.9	2423.7	28	1892.2	1967.2	2728.1	2873.5	18	2220.9	2353.3	1789.3	1969.4	2922.7	3155.7
	35	2590.0	2539.5	46	2097.9	2249.3	3044.2	3309.2	35	2578.4	2550.9	1771.2	2092.3	3101.2	3483.7
	36	2843.5	2865.4	84	2186.2	2339.6	3456.9	3588.3	75	2633.3	2640.2	2016.6	2151.7	3208.4	3291.5
	37	3045.8	3045.8	200	2196.5	2496.2	3645.3	3870.1	175	2950.9	2961.9	2263.7	2438.2	3529.1	3790.9
	38	3308.8	3258.3	562	2636.4	2804.5	3855.1	3981.2	491	3128.3	3141.4	2514.5	2632.1	3650.7	3787.8
	39	3397.8		1360					1138	3292.6	3292.6	2599.9	2725.9	3838.3	4006.2
	40	3546.3	3546.3	1677	2866.8	3015.4	4098.4	4268.3	1608	3391.5	3406.6	2725.9	2878.3	3956.0	4082.8
	41	3647.4	3647.4	1045	2949.2	3080.1	4214.6	4389.2	986	3473.5	3484.3	2793.9	2966.5	4045.3	4217.9
	42	3570.9	3582.5	117	2744.2	2904.9	4183.4	4328.8	133	3458.2	3469.1	2793.7	2946.2	3991.9	4209.8

Table 9.5   Difference between empirical and estimated percentiles of birthweight in gestation/sex/parity cells

Standards with only height known (*N* = 17 528)

| | Boys | | | | | | | Girls | | | | | | |
| | | | | Difference between actual and estimated — Percentile | | | | | | | Differnece between actual and estimated — Percentile | | | |
Weeks of gestation and parity	Mean	Difference between median + mean	N	5th	10th	90th	95th	Mean	Difference between median + mean	N	5th	10th	90th	95th
Para 0														
32	1843.1	41.2	13	3.9	4.0	19.2	0.0	1790.0	−69.6	8	—	26.7	−101.7	—
33	2134.6	58.3	13	−40.9	61.4	−37.0	−36.8	1976.5	−89.6	17	−132.6	−55.5	−34.0	−25.3
34	2360.3	69.2	32	112.7	334.6	−215.1	133.7	2133.8	10.3	21	91.5	−34.7	−0.3	−19.4
35	2489.8	29.0	44	102.6	−54.0	28.7	100.5	2314.1	−48.1	34	−118.2	−71.7	132.9	29.4
36	2701.2	−10.7	77	61.6	−39.8	−45.8	−61.5	2657.3	7.6	82	17.0	−48.1	−41.1	−17.0
37	2927.9	−34.8	169	−65.3	5.1	38.4	−21.6	2731.0	17.5	143	−28.9	−88.6	−54.8	−71.1
38	3177.5	10.0	392	21.1	−34.6	7.9	39.3	3021.8	10.3	346	−19.8	−35.7	35.7	19.8
39	3302.6	−17.2	901	−19.8	−36.5	−6.3	−65.7	3165.1	−10.5	832	−61.6	−35.8	14.8	−22.6
40	3420.5	−6.9	1345	22.3	6.2	−6.1	−1.5	3287.9	−10.0	1286	−18.5	−14.0	13.8	18.3
41	3508.2	−27.7	854	−60.9	−35.4	−6.2	−64.0	3379.6	−9.9	864	−57.7	−33.6	−5.7	−21
42	3475.0	−67.9	111	−46.6	−18.3	−15.7	54.1	3340.5	−15.9	121	−371.5	−427.8	−408.6	−425.1
Para 1+														
32	1970.0	−94.3	5	—	11.3	51.5	—	1902.5	−72.3	8	—	−13.6	−48.9	—
33	2126.9	0.0	16	−52.4	20.9	−7.7	−11.2	1970.6	39.8	16	48.8	67.3	19.5	—
34	2382.9	40.8	28	33.9	59.1	11.4	−33.8	2353.3	−132.4	18	−108.5	−141.1	−44.4	−129.9
35	2590.0	−50.5	46	−137.6	−150.9	37.4	−89.5	2550.9	27.5	35	14.0	−139.1	47.4	−166.8
36	2843.5	21.9	84	−68.0	−62.3	47.2	−19.5	2640.2	−6.9	75	−65.2	−49.2	−30.5	37.5
37	3045.8	0.0	200	25.2	−93.7	43.8	−0.2	2961.9	−11.0	175	−21.9	−38.4	−5.2	−109
38	3308.8	−50.5	562	−19.7	−36.0	−6.0	19.7	3141.4	−13.1	491	−25.5	−1.5	−12.5	−8.0
39	3397.8	—	1360	—	—	—	—	3292.6	0.0	1138	1.8	27.3	−6.4	22.7
40	3546.3	0.0	1677	−19.5	−14.8	−6.5	−23.0	3406.6	−15.1	1608	−15.0	−14.8	−6.3	19.5
41	3647.4	0.0	1045	−20.3	6.5	−6.4	−23.4	3484.3	−10.8	986	−20	−36.7	−6.5	−23.2
42	3570.9	11.6	117	67.1	73.0	−20.5	0.7	3469.1	−10.9	133	−44.3	−38.9	39.0	−21.0

Table 9.6 Empirical percentages falling into the estimated 5th, 10th and 90th percentiles in gestation/sex/parity cells
Standards with only height known (N = 17 528)

	Weeks of gestation and parity	Boys							Girls						
					Actual %							Actual %			
		Mean	Range	N	Under 5%	Under 10%	Over 90%	Over 95%	Mean	Range	N	Under 5%	Under 10%	Over 90%	Over 95%
Para 0	32	1843.1	1113.1	13	4.2	6.2	9.3	4.9	1790.0	1531.7	8	–	6.6	13.8	-2.2
	33	2134.6	1143.8	13	–	12.7	11.5	5.5	1976.5	1701.3	17	–	6.5	12.5	7.5
	34	2360.3	2026.4	32	9.1	21.2	18.1	–	2133.8	1586.4	21	7.1	9.4	9.6	5.4
	35	2489.8	1827.8	44	6.2	8.4	8.1	1.4	2314.1	2623.7	34	3.6	5.9	6.5	4.6
	36	2701.2	2141.8	77	6.4	8.2	11.1	8.4	2657.3	1604.7	82	5.4	8.4	13.2	6.3
	37	2927.9	2477.4	169	3.5	10.8	9.1	5.5	2731.0	2122.6	143	3.6	6.9	12.5	6.6
	38	3177.5	2532.5	392	5.5	7.7	9.4	3.5	3021.8	3091.9	346	4.5	8.2	9.1	4.5
	39	3302.6	3000.0	901	4.5	9.1	10.1	5.5	3165.1	3701.0	832	4.5	8.3	9.3	5.5
	40	3420.5	2858.2	1345	5.5	10.1	10.7	4.9	3287.9	2877.7	1286	4.5	9.3	10.3	4.5
	41	3508.2	2746.2	854	3.5	8.3	11.3	6.5	3379.6	2950.0	864	3.5	8.3	10.3	5.5
	42	3475.0	2671.4	111	3.8	9.2	11.7	3.9	3340.5	2301.3	121	–	–	39.2	25.1
Para 1+	32	1970.0	942.6	5	–	–	12.3	–	1902.5	922	8	–	9.3	13.9	6.6
	33	2126.9	1151.9	16	–	12.1	11.5	6.4	1970.6	1022.8	16	7.5	15.4	8.9	–
	34	2382.9	1117.6	28	7.5	12.9	8.9	5.9	2353.3	1588.8	18	3.1	5.7	11.3	7.3
	35	2590.0	2157.5	46	3.2	5.1	9.6	9.2	2550.9	2384.7	35	4.1	6.3	9.4	7.2
	36	2843.5	2409.9	84	4.2	7.2	11.5	5.7	2640.2	2286.7	75	3.9	7.1	12.1	3.7
	37	3045.8	3796.9	200	5.3	7.2	9.1	5.2	2961.9	2618.3	175	4.5	9.1	10.1	7.5
	38	3308.8	3361.9	562	4.5	9.1	11.2	4.5	3141.4	2507.4	491	4.4	9.9	10.3	5.4
	39	3397.8		1360					3292.6	2938.5	1138	4.1	11.2	10.3	5.5
	40	3546.3	3142.8	1677	4.5	9.3	10.2	5.2	3406.6	2873.9	1608	5.1	9.3	11.3	4.5
	41	3647.4	2923.6	1045	4.5	10.3	10.1	5.5	3484.3	3193.3	986	4.5	9.1	10.3	5.5
	42	3570.9	2342.5	117	6.9	11.1	10.7	4.3	3469.1	2265.8	133	3.5	8.2	9.6	6.0

size. Taking the problem of the systematic departures from normality seriously would entail the estimation of such standards from the distribution of birthweights in gestation/sex/parity/maternal height/maternal weight cells, a literally impossible task for the derivation of local standards. The techniques of statistical modelling which are presently available do not permit of a sensitive adjustment for discrete forms of the distribution of birthweight within each gestation/sex/parity cell in the estimation of coefficients for maternal size.

More generally, the distributions observed in this study are specific not only to a particular location, but also to a particular sample and this, too, has implications for the clinical use of standards. For reasons which have been discussed at some length (see chapter 5), the sample has included only 'certain' gestations. The utility of standardised birthweight in the assessment of babies where the gestation is less than certain is dubious. Furthermore, the distributions of birthweight to which standards refer relate to a particular epoch and may not apply precisely to babies born subsequently. Although regular monitoring and updating of local standards may minimise the imprecisions introduced in this way they continue to represent a difficulty.

Overall, then, birthweight standards cannot be considered as a precise clinical tool. The apparent exactness of the criteria of 'light', or 'heavy for dates' is deceptive and it is incumbent upon clinicians not to be deceived. This is especially important at the pre-term weeks (see above and chapter 12 for further discussion). On the other hand, standards do provide some sense of the relative appropriateness of the baby's weight to its gestational age and, at present, they represent the best possible way of gaining such a sense. Their intelligent use, in the knowledge of their status, still has a part to play in the neonatal paediatrician's task of assessing babies.

10

The Relationship between Social Class and Standardised Birthweight Scores

INTRODUCTION

The association between social class and birthweight has been noted in a number of birthweight surveys. Butler and Alberman (1969) for example, showed that babies born to mothers of the highest social class (1) were on average 110 grams heavier than those born to mothers of social class V and that the percentage of low birthweight babies (< 2500 grams) rose from 4.9% to 8.2% between highest and lowest social classes (their pages 52-53). For babies born after 36 weeks gestation, the differences between social classes I and II and social classes IV and V were significant at each week of gestation (their pages 60-62). Both social class and the interaction between social class and gestation had significant effects on birthweight in an analysis of variance including only gestation and social class as independent variables (their pages 58-59), but not in a more complex model which also included age, parity, smoking, pre-eclampsia and height (their page 66). It is obviously an important and interesting issue which can and should be further explored in our data.

A more recent attempt to assess the effect of socio-economic status on birthweight is that by Dowding (1981). Unfortunately, although she has a large quantity of apparently excellent data, her treatment of them leaves much to be desired. It might occasionally be legitimate to treat 'social group' as an interval variable as a presentational device as she does in her figure 2. But it is nonsense to calculate a 'mean social group number' as she does in a vain attempt to differentiate between the effects of birth order and parity. The attempt would, in any case, be vain because her 'analysis' is in terms of the percentage of the different weight categories born to each social group. We cannot sort out the complex interactions of socio-economic status with other factors (in the determination of birthweight) on the basis of just three sets of eight observations.

In the Aberdeen data the relation of social class to raw birthweight follows a

133

similar pattern to that noted by Butler and Alberman (1969) and many others: equally, there are complex problems of estimating the 'true' effect of social class on birthweight because of the labyrinthine nature of the interrelationship between social class and nearly everything else. Some of the complexities, viz. the non-linear effects of 'normal' factors such as gestation and parity, can be avoided by the use of standardised birthweight scores such as those developed in chapters 7 and 8. Indeed, another purpose of including this analysis in the book is to illustrate the usefulness of the standards that have been developed.

This is especially important as the use of birthweight standards for research purposes depends upon the presumption of equivalent birthweight distributions within each sex/parity/gestation cell (see the concluding chapter for further discussion). This chapter, then, explores the effects of social class on standardised birthweight scores in the light of the effects of maternal height, maternal weight for height (z weight) and her smoking habits during pregnancy.

MATERIALS

The analyses to be presented are based on the two different samples:

(1) Where height is the only parameter of maternal size used, the analyses are based on the standards sample excluding those with missing data for social class or for smoking habits ($N = 14\,197$);

(2) the analyses including maternal weight are based on a subsample for whom weights are available. Because the effects of maternal z weight on birthweight are only apparent among term babies the sample is further restricted to those with gestations over 36 weeks ($N = 3756$).

Both these samples are restricted to married women only. Note also that the distributions of smoking and social class are different in the two samples (see chapter 6). Whilst this might have influenced the estimated coefficients, pre-liminary analyses suggested that this was not a significant problem.

The standardised birthweight score used in the ensuing analyses as the dependent variable is that presented at the beginning of chapter 8 without corrections for maternal size. Separate standardised birthweight scores (SBS) have been calculated for the subsample for whom maternal mid-term weights are available and for the whole standards sample. While the differences are minimal, the score used is the one appropriate to the sample being analysed. Social class and smoking variables are those described in chapter 6.

Some commentary is necessary on the nature of these latter two variables which have not previously been discussed in detail.

Occupationally derived social class (Registrar General, 1981)

This, in which a woman's class is defined in terms of her husband's occupation, is an apt way of displaying gradients of socially differentiated health outcomes, but of itself, has little explanatory power (cf. DHSS, 1980). While it may indicate broad differences in life-style it falls short of identifying the causes of divergence in outcome. Moreover, some studies have shown that variations in birthweight within a broad social class grouping can be related to other behavioural/cultural variables (see, for example, Illsley and Mitchell, 1984). It is, however, generally recognised as the best broad indicator of socio-economic status.

The smoking variable

As explained in chapter 6, this is a categorisation of self-reported consumption figures. Not only are self-reported data notoriously unreliable, but also it seems probable that there will be social class differences in mis-reporting.

ANALYSES OF THE EFFECTS OF MATERNAL HEIGHT, z WEIGHT, SMOKING AND SOCIAL CLASS ON STANDARDISED BIRTHWEIGHT SCORES

Table 10.1 shows the mean and standard deviations of standardised birthweight score for the different social classes. The gradient, equivalent to about 75 grams from highest to lowest social classes represents, as it were, the problem posed to this chapter.

Table 10.1   Mean standard deviation – SBS
by social class

Social class	Mean	SBS SD	N
I and II	0.097	0.96	4241
IIIn	0.063	0.95	1355
IIIm	−0.019	1.01	4959
IV and V	−0.086	1.03	3642

eta = 0.07; eta² = 0.005.

It is difficult to suggest *a priori* model specifications for the analysis. It seems reasonable to suggest that 'classness' (whatever that means) influences women's size and their tendency to smoke rather than the alternative suggestion that size and smoking determine 'classness' in some way. Unfortunately, the problem is, in practice, made more complicated because our measure of 'classness' is based on the husband's occupation: and both adult height certainly does, and smoking habits might, precede marriage. The direction of causality when using the usual social class variable as a measure of 'classness' is therefore not so clear.

For a woman's height and smoking habits might have influenced her choice or possibility of partner.

Our approach to this problem using standardised birthweight scores is to perform the analyses under a variety of different hierarchical model specifications. The differences in the effects provide some insight into the non-orthogonality of the independent variables in terms of their effect upon standardised birthweight scores. Particular attention is also paid to the interaction term in each of the analyses.

However, even if there were no conceptual difficulties of this kind, there would remain a problem in interpreting the results of these various analyses because of the statistical associations between social class (however measured), maternal size and smoking habits. These are illustrated in the Aberdeen data in figures 10.1 and 10.2. Figure 10.1 shows that heavier smoking is associated with lower social class; figure 10.2 shows both that maternal height decreases and that maternal weight-for-height increases with decreasing social class. It cannot, therefore, be conclusively determined which variable is representing which real effect: we return briefly to this problem in the discussion chapter.

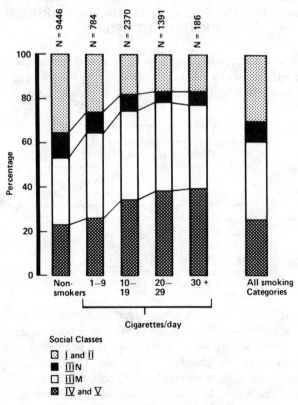

Figure 10.1   Social class by smoking

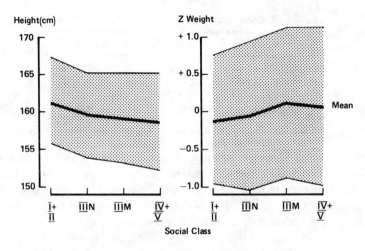

Figure 10.2   Social class by maternal size

The effects of maternal height

In analyses in which height is the only parameter of maternal size used, it consistently accounts for the highest proportion of the sums of squares of all the independent variables no matter in which position it enters the model (table 10.2). As table 10.2 also shows, the slope of the regression line (the estimate coefficient) does not vary with its position in the model.

Table 10.2   The effects of height on SBS under different model specifications

	eta^2	*F*	Coefficient
(1) Enters model first	0.055	866.94	0.037
(2) Enters after social class	0.052	812.07	0.037
(3) Enters after smoking	0.050	781.97	0.037
(4) Enters after both social class and smoking	0.050	768.34	0.037

When maternal height is included as a covariate in a model including maternal z weight, it accounts for a similar proportion of the sum of squares to the proportion accounted for when it is the sole parameter of maternal size used (eta^2 = 0.053) and its coefficient is slightly, but not significantly reduced (0.036 SBS/cm).

The effects of maternal height do, however, vary within smoking categories: the coefficients are shown in table 10.3. The interaction term (after main effects) is significant ($F = 3.13, p < 0.05$) and the effect of the interaction, on the whole, is that the regression line for maternal height becomes steeper as

Table 10.3 Coefficients for height by smoking categories

Cigarettes per day	Coefficient	Standard error
0	0.0347	0.0015
1–9	0.0379	0.0058
10–19	0.0374	0.0033
20–29	0.0472	0.0042
30+	0.0436	0.0085

smoking increases. However, when the interaction term is included in a model which incorporates the effects of maternal z weight, it is no longer significant ($F = 1.0$). This suggests that the observed differences in the estimated slope of the regression of standardised birthweight score on maternal height are related to differences in maternal z weight within the various categories of smoking.

The effects of maternal height do vary slightly within social class categories with the slope of the regression increasing with lower social class. But the term representing this interaction is never significant under any model specification.

The effects of maternal z weight

Table 10.4 shows the analysis of the effects of maternal z weight on standardised birthweight score in a similar way to those presented for maternal height. As with maternal height, maternal z weight consistently explains the largest proportion of the sums of squares under each of the model specifications. Although the eta^2 does vary with the position in the model, the differences are not significant and the slope of the regression line does not change.

Table 10.4 The effects of maternal z weight on SBS under different model specifications

		eta^2	F	Coefficient
(1)	Enters model first	0.068	241.48	0.0026
(2)	Enters model after social class	0.071	254.38	0.0026
(3)	Enters model after smoking	0.066	237.54	0.0026
(4)	Enters model after both social class and smoking	0.068	240.51	0.0026

The effects of maternal z weight do vary within smoking categories, as is shown in table 10.5. The interaction term for the effects of maternal weight-for-height and smoking on standardised birthweight score is significant ($F = 2.87$, $p < 0.05$) after the main effects of the other independent variables, and remains significant in the model in which maternal height and maternal z weight both enter the analysis ($F = 2.59$, $p < 0.05$). The effect of the interaction is such that, among smokers, increments in standardised birthweight score associated with maternal z weight increases until the level of 20–29 cigarettes/day is

Table 10.5 Coefficients for z weight by smoking categories

Cigarettes per day	Coefficient	Standard error
0	0.0025	0.0002
1–9	0.0023	0.0007
10–19	0.0026	0.0004
20–29	0.0038	0.0004
30+	0.0010	0.0010

reached. Among women who smoke 30 or more cigarettes per day, the effect of differences in maternal weight for height on SBS is not significant. Of course, the standard error of this coefficient is large because the number in this category in this sample is relatively small ($N = 63$) but this does not account for the substantially smaller coefficients.

Although the coefficients for maternal z weight do differ within social class, neither the differences between social class categories nor the corresponding interaction terms are significant.

The effects of smoking

In models including maternal height as the only parameter of maternal size, the proportion of the sums of squares explained by smoking differs with its position in the model, decreasing after either maternal height or social class enter the analysis (table 10.6). Table 10.6 also shows that the proportions of the sums of squares explained by smoking varies according to its position in models including the effects of maternal z weight in the subsample for whom maternal weight data are available. Although these variations in the effects of smoking are not significant, they do reflect the fact that smoking is not orthogonal to maternal height, z weight and social class.

The parameter estimates for the effects of smoking also vary slightly with the position of smoking in the model, although the differences between the four hierarchical specifications are not significant. The general pattern for the effects of smoking is that increased consumption is associated with decreasing standardised birthweight scores. The effects are not, however, linear, the largest decrement being associated with the change from smoking less than 10 cigarettes per day to smoking between 10 and 19 cigarettes per day. The decrease in standardised birthweight score associated with smoking 30 or more cigarettes per day is generally less than that associated with smoking 20-29 cigarettes per day, especially in the subpopulation for whom maternal weight data are available.

In the sample as a whole, the effects of smoking do vary with social class. Table 10.7 shows the parameter estimates for smoking within social class categories. The interaction term accounts for a significant proportion of the sum of squares after the main effects ($F = 3.25, p < 0.05$) and the differences between these parameter estimates for smoking and the estimates for the sample as a

Table 10.6   Effects of smoking on SBS under different model specifications

(a) Height only models

	eta^2	F	0	1–9	10–19	20–29	30+
(1) Enters model first	0.042	148.59	0.304	0.151	−0.073	−0.197	−0.185
(2) Enters after height	0.037	142.71	0.297	0.135	−0.051	−0.187	−0.194
(3) Enters after social class	0.038	141.55	0.303	0.149	−0.075	−0.213	−0.164
(4) Enters after both height and social class	0.035	124.05	0.304	0.151	−0.073	−0.197	−0.185

(b) Weight only models

	eta^2	F	0	1–9	10–19	20–29	30+
(1) Enters model first	0.034	32.75	0.253	0.145	−0.091	−0.227	−0.080
(2) Enters after weight	0.033	31.25	0.263	0.138	−0.033	−0.203	−0.165
(3) Enters after social class	0.032	30.04	0.253	0.143	−0.092	−0.235	−0.069
(4) Enters after both weight and social class	0.029	27.22	0.253	0.145	−0.091	−0.277	−0.080

(c) Height and weight

	eta^2	F	0	1–9	10–19	20–29	30+
(1) Enters after height and weight	0.029	27.30	0.242	0.133	−0.091	−0.228	−0.056
(2) Enters after height, weight and social class	0.027	25.70	0.242	0.133	−0.091	−0.228	−0.056

Table 10.7   Parameter estimates for the effects of smoking within social class

Social class	Cigarettes per day				
	0	1–9	10–19	20–29	30+
I and II	0.273	0.072*	0.010*	−0.102*	−0.253*
IIIn	0.279	0.119	−0.014*	−0.210	−0.174
IIIm	0.313	0.195*	−0.121*	−0.208	−0.179
IV and V	0.438*	0.314*	−0.156	−0.391*	−0.205

*Differs significantly ($p < 0.05$) from sample estimates.

whole are significant where indicated. With the exception of social classes I and II, the deleterious effect of smoking more than 29 cigarettes per day is less than the effect associated with smoking 20-29 cigarettes per day. For social classes I and II the transition from not smoking to smoking 1-9 cigarettes per day has the most marked effect.

The effect of the interaction upon standardised birthweight scores is substantial: the difference between the effects of not smoking and of smoking 20-29 cigarettes per day varies from a minimum of 0.489 SBS for social class IIIn to a maximum of 0.829 SBS for social classes IV and V. But, it seems important to stress that the figures for consumption are self-reported and the differences especially in the size of the decrement associated with the difference between not smoking and smoking 1-9 cigarettes per day may reflect class differentiated reporting style. Furthermore, this interaction effect is not significant in the subpopulation for whom maternal weight is available ($F = 1.34$) which may suggest that maternal weight differences between social classes explain the observed differences in the effects of smoking. (This point is also considered in the next chapter.)

The effects of social class

As table 10.8 shows, the effects of social class are small under all model specifications. In analyses in which maternal height is the only parameter of maternal size, social class explains a significant proportion of the sums of squares in models in which it enters first or second but, even in these models, the parameter estimates do not differ significantly from zero. Social class never has a significant F ratio when it enters any of the analyses after either or both of the parameters of maternal size and smoking.

In the subpopulation for whom maternal weight data are available, social class becomes insignificant when entered after smoking, although the effect of adjusting for the covariance of maternal z weight with standardised birthweight score is to increase the proportion of variance explained by social class. Moreover, in that model, the estimates for the parameters of highest and lowest social classes are significantly different from the overall sample values.

THE COMPLETE ANALYSIS OF VARIANCE

Table 10.9 presents the analysis of variance of standardised birthweight scores for the subsample for whom maternal weight data are available. Maternal height and z weight together account for 11.9% of the variance in standardised birthweight scores. Under a variety of model specifications, the coefficients for maternal height and z weight do not vary significantly. Smoking then accounts for a further 2.7% of the variance in standardised birthweight scores. Overall, the decrease in standardised birthweight scores associated with smoking 20-29

Table 10.8   Effects of social class on SBS under different model specifications

(a) Height only models

		eta²	F	I and II	IIIn	IIIm	IV and V
(1)	Enters model first	0.005	24.56*	−0.014	0.016	0.012	−0.014
(2)	Enters after height	0.002	8.03*	−0.006	0.024	0.009	−0.027
(3)	Enters after smoking	0.001	3.98*	0.340	0.291	−0.167	−0.464
(4)	Enters after both height and smoking	0.000	0.094	−1.060	0.833	0.949	0.722

(b) Weight only models

		eta²	F	I and II	IIIn	IIIm	IV and V
(1)	Enters model first	0.003	3.31*	0.052	0.026	−0.033	−0.045
(2)	Enters after weight	0.006	7.66*	0.067*	0.032	−0.036	−0.064*
(3)	Enters after smoking	0.000	0.035	0.056*	0.023	−0.033	−0.046
(4)	Enters after both weight and smoking	0.002	1.98	0.052	0.026	−0.033	−0.045

(c) Height and weight models

		eta²	F	I and II	IIIn	IIIm	IV and V
(1)	Enters after height and weight	0.002	2.73*	0.025	0.015	−0.024	−0.016
(2)	Enters after height, weight and smoking	0.000	0.17	0.025	0.015	−0.0014	−0.026

*Significant ($p < 0.05$).

Table 10.9   Analyses of variance − 'best fit' model

	Sum of squares	Degree of freedom	F
z Weight	241.48	1	283.51
Height	203.11	1	238.46
Smoking	102.80	4	30.17
z Weight by smoking	8.84	4	2.59
	3196.57		
Total SS	3752.80		

cigarettes per day against not smoking is 0.5 SBS, that is roughly equivalent to 200 grams in birthweight.

The interaction between maternal smoking and z weight is significant. For those who smoke 20 cigarettes or more per day, increasing weight is associated with a greater increment in standardised birthweight score than for non-smokers or those who smoke less than 20 cigarettes per day after adjusting for the preceding main effects and interactions. This would seem to contradict Hawarth *et al.*'s (1980) report that maternal obesity and smoking have independent effects and may indirectly relate to Papoz *et al.*'s (1982) findings which suggest an enhanced effect of nutritional differences among smokers. As chapter 11 will show, however, differences in the incidence of pre-eclampsia play their part in the observed pattern.

The analyses presented above show that the 'effects' of social class are never large and can be accounted for by either parameter of maternal size together with smoking. Table 10.10 shows the mean standardised birthweight scores

Table 10.10 Mean SBS adjusted for height and z weight and the interaction of z weight and smoking by social class and smoking

Social class	Cigarettes per day									
	0		1–9		10–19		20–29		30+	
	N	Mean	N	Mean	N	Mean	N	Mean	N	Mean
I and II	3364	0.14	202	0.00	418	−0.20	226	−0.22	31	−0.12
IIIn	1025	0.11	71	0.04	175	−0.10	73	−0.22	11	−0.23
IIIm	3061	0.13	306	−0.02	961	−0.25	561	−0.38	70	−0.23
IV and V	2016	0.14	205	−0.02	816	−0.28	531	−0.42	74	−0.23

adjusted for maternal height, z weight and their interaction (cf. chapter 8) in smoking and social class categories. Although the eye of faith may detect a social class gradient among women who smoke between 10 and 29 cigarettes per day none of the means differ significantly from the overall mean for the smoking category. Essentially, the social class gradient in mean corrected standardised birthweight score can be accounted for by factors of maternal size and smoking.

EPILOGUE

However, this finding does not represent a final statement about the effects of social class on birthweight. Using standardised birthweight scores corrected for maternal size, it is possible to ask whether the proportions of babies with standardised birthweight scores below the notional criteria of −1.282 SBS (the

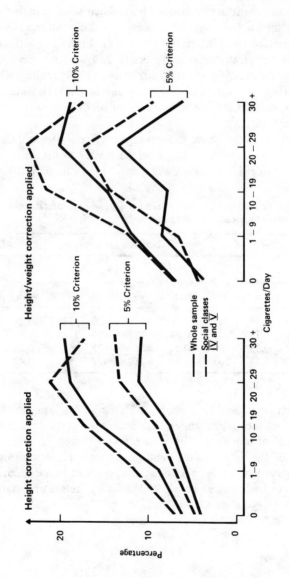

Figure 10.3 Percentage of light-for-dates babies by smoking categories: sample values — for social classes IV and V

normal equivalent 10th percentile) and -1.645 SBS (the normal equivalent 5th percentile) differ by social class. This procedure does make corrections for maternal size easily possible although there is the problem of non-normality of the distributions of birthweight in gestation/sex/parity groups (see chapter 9). Whilst the groups so defined are 'light for dates', we recall that this is not equivalent to a clinical diagnosis of growth retardation (see chapters 5 and 7).

The distribution of standardised birthweight scores after adjusting for maternal height or for maternal height and z weight within cells defined by smoking and social class is such that, although the means do not differ significantly by social class, the proportion of babies falling below -1.282 SBS and -1.645 SBS do differ. Figure 10.3 shows the proportion of 'light for dates' babies born to mothers of social classes IV and V compared to the overall sample values within smoking categories. The differences are always significant (two-tailed p on 't' test for differences in proportions < 0.05) among women who smoke between 10 and 29 cigarettes per day. The social class gradient is such that, for women smoking 10–19 cigarettes per day the proportion of 'light for dates' babies in social class IV and V is three times the proportion in social class I and II (14.2% against 3.7%) using the notional 5th percentile as a criterion and more than double (21.9% against 10.2%) using the notional 10th percentile as a criterion. For over a quarter of the sample who smoke between 10 and 29 cigarettes per day differing social class is associated with significant differences in their prospects of giving birth to a 'light for dates' baby.

This finding is similar to that noted by Miller and Hassanein (1976: 57) and further suggests some support for Yerushalmy's (1972) controversial argument that the characteristics of the smoker other than her smoking play their part in the higher incidence of low birthweight among smokers.

11

Pre-eclampsia, smoking and standardised birthweight

INTRODUCTION

This chapter is concerned primarily to assess the effects of pre-eclampsia on standardised birthweight scores taking into account the joint variation with smoking habits.

Proteinuric pre-eclampsia (moderate and severe pre-eclampsia in the definitions given in chapter 5) has an incidence of 4.1% in the Aberdeen sample. As such, it represents by far the most common pregnancy-associated maternal disease which affects birthweight. It has been known for some time that pre-eclampsia is less common among smokers than among non-smokers (see e.g. Duffus and MacGillivray, 1968; Butler and Alberman, 1969) and this finding is replicated in the Aberdeen sample. Figure 11.1 shows the incidence of pre-eclampsia by smoking categories. While the incidence of 'mild' (non-proteinuric) pre-eclampsia increases with increasing cigarette consumption, it is only among the heaviest smokers (those who smoke more than 29 cigarettes per day) that the incidence approaches that for non-smokers. Among those who smoke less than 30 cigarettes per day the incidence of proteinuric pre-eclampsia decreases with increasing cigarette consumption.

These incidence figures, suggesting an antagonistic relationship between smoking and pre-eclampsia, indicate that the assessment of their joint effects on birthweight is likely to be of particular interest. The intention of this chapter is to use the standardised birthweight scores developed in chapter 8 to estimate and assess the effects of pre-eclampsia on birthweight and, in particular, to discuss the joint effects of smoking and pre-eclampsia.

MATERIALS AND METHODS

The data analysed are based on the sample used to derive standardised birthweight scores, excluding those for whom data on smoking habits and pre-eclamp-

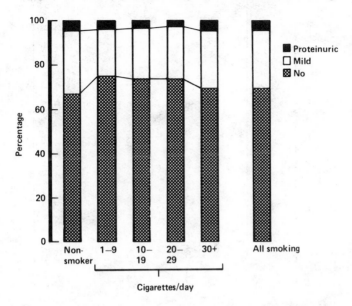

Figure 11.1   Pre-eclampsia by smoking categories

sia are missing. There were 16 869 cases with complete smoking and pre-eclampsia data and of these 4772 were weighed between 18 and 22 weeks gestation. The definitions of pre-eclampsia were given in chapter 6 and, for these analyses, 'moderate' and 'severe' pre-eclampsia have been combined to give a class of 'proteinuric pre-eclampsia'.

As in the previous chapter, we have problems of model specification and of multicollinearity. In principle, maternal height and weight precede the likelihood of contracting pre-eclampsia. However, the preceding chapter has shown that, in assessing the joint effects of maternal smoking and pre-eclampsia on birthweight, this presumption is doubtful in the case of smoking and maternal weight. In addition, for multiparae, it is difficult to be sanguine about the effects of hypertensive stress and treatment in first pregnancy upon subsequent diet and therefore maternal weight. We shall, however, take it as axiomatic in the ensuing analysis that the effects of smoking and of pre-eclampsia should be assessed after those of maternal size, thereby simplifying the analytic task considerably.

Nevertheless, there remains the problem that the incidence of pre-eclampsia varies with the factors that are controlled for in standardised birthweight scores. As table 11.1 shows, mild pre-eclampsia is more common among women who deliver after 36 weeks gestation while the incidence of proteinuric pre-eclampsia is higher among those who deliver pre-term. This latter finding may, of course, reflect the more active management of more severely affected pregnancies. The induction rate for those with proteinuric pre-eclampsia pre-term is 76.1% compared to an overall induction rate pre-term of 26.0%. The proteinuric groups

Table 11.1 Incidence of pre-eclampsia by gestation (pre-term/term), sex and parity (0, 1+)

Parity 0

	Pre-eclampsia						
	None		Mild		Prot.		All
	N	%	N	%	N	%	N
Boys, 0							
Pre-term	103	60.2	33	19.3	35	20.5	171
Term	2078	58.0	1271	35.5	234	6.5	3583
All	2181	58.1	1304	34.7	269	7.2	3754
Girls, 0							
Pre-term	87	54.7	35	22.0	37	23.3	159
Term	2079	60.8	1128	33.0	210	6.1	3417
All	2166	60.6	1163	32.5	247	6.9	3576
Both sexes para, 0							
Pre-term	190	57.6	68	20.6	72	21.8	330
Term	4157	59.4	2399	34.3	444	6.3	7000
All	4347	59.3	2467	33.7	516	7.0	7330

Parity 1+

	Pre-eclampsia						
	None		Mild		Prot.		All
	N	%	N	%	N	%	N
Boys, 1+							
Pre-term	134	77.0	29	16.7	11	6.3	174
Term	3735	77.3	1023	21.2	74	1.5	4832
All	3869	77.3	1052	21.0	85	1.7	5006
Girls, 1+							
Pre-term	112	75.7	27	18.2	9	6.1	148
Term	3410	77.8	896	20.4	79	1.8	4385
All	3522	77.7	923	20.4	88	1.9	4533
Both sexes para, 1+							
Pre-term	246	76.4	56	17.4	20	6.2	322
Term	7145	77.5	1919	20.8	153	1.7	9217
All	7391	77.5	1975	20.7	173	1.8	9539

All para

	Pre-eclampsia						
	None		Mild		Prot.		All
	N	%	N	%	N	%	N
All para, Boys							
Pre-term	237	68.7	62	18.0	46	13.3	345
Term	5813	69.1	2294	27.3	308	3.7	8415
All	6050	69.1	2356	26.9	354	4.0	8760
All para, Girls							
Pre-term	199	64.8	62	20.2	46	15.0	307
Term	5489	70.4	2024	25.9	289	3.7	7802
All	5688	70.1	2086	25.7	335	4.1	8109
All							
Pre-term	436	66.9	124	19.0	92	14.1	652
Term	11302	69.7	4318	26.6	597	3.7	16217
All	11738	69.6	4442	26.3	689	4.1	16869

form 40.2% of all pre-term inductions. Overall, pre-eclampsia is more common among women bearing boys than among women bearing girls (see also Campbell *et al.*, 1983b) and more common among primiparae than among multiparae.

Table 11.2 shows the mean maternal height and z weights (weight-for-height index) for the sample by smoking and pre-eclampsia categories. Although the differences in maternal height are slight, women who smoke tend to be shorter than those who do not smoke and women who develop proteinuric pre-eclampsia tend to be shorter than those who are normotensive or who develop hypertension without proteinuria. Normotensive women were on average lighter for their

Table 11.2   Maternal size by smoking and pre-eclampsia categories

Cigarettes per day	Pre-eclampsia							
	None mean	*N*	Mild mean	*N*	Proteinuric mean	*N*	All mean	*N*
(a) Mean height (cm)								
0	159.90	6987	160.01	3006	158.89	472	159.89	10465
−9	159.39	1603	159.86	445	158.98	80	159.47	2128
−19	159.26	1867	159.48	579	158.76	83	159.29	2529
−29	158.88	1124	159.64	353	158.50	44	159.05	1521
30+	159.12	157	159.20	59	156.50	10	159.02	226
All	159.62	11738	159.88	4442	158.82	689	159.66	16869
(b) Mean z-weight								
0	−0.10	1988	0.19	936	0.13	160	0.00	3084
−9	−0.03	187	−0.07	73	0.69	15	0.00	275
−19	−0.16	573	0.21	197	0.21	34	−0.05	804
−29	−0.10	379	0.32	120	0.60	19	0.02	518
30+	−0.20	62	0.59	24	0.71	5	0.06	91
All	−0.10	3189	0.20	1350	0.23	233	0.00	4772

height than those who develop pre-eclampsia of either variety. It has been suggested that this may be due to the early effects of the disorder (Vedra and Pavlikova, 1969). On the whole, among normotensive women, increasing cigarette consumption is associated with declining mean z weight, whilst this pattern is reversed for both classes of pre-eclampsia where increased consumption tends to be associated with an increasing weight-for height index.

These empirical intercorrelations cannot, of course, be avoided but they must, therefore, inform the interpretations of any results. Furthermore, whatever the results from the multivariate analysis, it becomes equally important to look in detail at the breakdown of the effects in cells defined by categories of pre-eclampsia and sex of infant, parity and gestation as well as being aware of the possible overlap in effect as between pre-eclampsia and maternal size and smoking habits.

Pre-eclampsia, smoking and standardised birthweight scores without corrections for maternal height and weight

In analysis of variance for the sample as a whole, smoking ($F = 176.25$, $p <$ 0.001), pre-eclampsia ($F = 14.63$, $p < 0.001$) and their interaction ($F = 3.34$, $p < 0.001$) account for significant proportions of the variance in standardised birthweight scores when no corrections are introduced for maternal height and weight.

Table 11.3 shows the mean standardised birthweight score in sex/parity groups for pre-eclampsia and smoking categories. The variation of standardised birthweight scores with smoking categories has been discussed in the previous chapter. The variation with category of pre-eclampsia is such that there is a small but consistent positive effect associated with mild pre-eclampsia and a consistent negative effect associated with proteinuric pre-eclampsia which is small amongst primiparae and larger amongst multiparae. There is no apparent variation with sex.

In the body of the table, the pattern is similar so that for each category of smoking, mild (non-proteinuric) pre-eclampsia is associated with the highest standardised birthweight score and proteinuric pre-eclampsia with the lowest standardised birthweight score. The few exceptions to the general pattern tend to occur amongst those who smoke and report smoking less than 20 cigarettes per day. In particular, for those who smoke between 10 and 19 cigarettes per day, in only one out of four cases is proteinuric pre-eclampsia associated with the *lowest* standardised birthweight score. Among normotensive women, increased cigarette consumption is associated with a consistent decrease.

Pre-eclampsia, smoking and standardised birthweight scores with corrections for maternal height and weight

We appear to have found a general pattern of effects on the basis of the uncorrected standardised birthweight scores. However, we have shown earlier that there are differences in maternal size, and especially in maternal weight, in categories defined by smoking and pre-eclampsia. It is, therefore, important to consider how the correction for maternal size affects the observed pattern. The analysis is conducted separately for term and for pre-term babies because the correction for maternal weight is only appropriate with term babies (see chapter 8).

CORRECTIONS FOR MATERNAL HEIGHT AND WEIGHT AMONG TERM BABIES

In the Aberdeen population, the subsample for whom maternal data are available and who delivered after 36 weeks gestation is only 4551. The division into categories defined by sex of infant, parity and pre-eclampsia renders 60 possible cells

Table 11.3 Mean standardised birthweight scores (without correction for maternal size) by smoking and pre-eclampsia categories in sex/parity (0, 1+) groups

Pre-eclampsia

Cigarettes per day	None mean	N	Mild mean	N	Prot. mean	N	All mean	N
Boys, 0								
0	0.12	1261	0.15	869	0.03	187	0.12	2317
–9	–0.14	340	0.16	136	–0.41	25	–0.07	501
–19	–0.34	366	–0.16	178	–0.20	36	–0.28	580
–29	–0.41	189	–0.21	109	–0.53	16	–0.35	314
30+	–0.03	25	0.05	12	–1.09	5	–0.13	42
All	–0.05	2181	0.08	1304	–0.10	269	–0.01	3754
Girls, 0								
0	0.12	1241	0.19	749	0.02	163	0.13	2153
–9	–0.11	354	–0.05	140	–0.05	42	–0.09	536
–19	–0.26	353	–0.18	167	–0.43	26	–0.25	546
–29	–0.42	196	–0.34	86	–0.51	15	–0.40	297
30+	–0.63	22	–0.17	21	1.17	1	–0.37	44
All	–0.04	2166	0.06	1163	–0.07	247	–0.01	3576

Pre-eclampsia

Cigarettes per day	None mean	N	Mild mean	N	Prot. mean	N	All mean	N
Boys, 1+								
0	0.16	2293	0.12	734	–0.36	65	0.14	3092
–9	–0.06	490	–0.09	97	–0.54	55	–0.07	592
–19	–0.29	650	–0.14	115	–0.02	8	–0.26	773
–29	–0.39	382	–0.27	94	–1.00	7	–0.37	483
30+	–0.50	54	–0.37	12	NA	NA	–0.47	66
All	0.00	3869	0.03	1052	–0.39	85	0.00	5006
Girls, 1+								
0	0.16	2192	0.13	654	–0.09	57	0.15	2903
–9	–0.09	419	–0.01	72	–0.09	8	–0.08	499
–19	–0.35	498	–0.08	119	–0.09	13	–0.29	630
–29	–0.44	357	–0.35	64	–1.43	6	–0.41	427
30+	–0.56	56	–0.30	14	–2.16	4	–0.60	74
All	–0.01	3522	0.05	923	–0.27	88	0.00	4533

(cf. table 11.3), some of which contain very small numbers or have no cases. For example, in this subsample there were no boys born to mothers who smoked between 1 and 9 cigarettes per day and who developed proteinuric pre-eclampsia. Even with a sample of 4551 there are severe constraints on analysis.

In analysis of variance, smoking ($F = 43.89$, $p < 0.001$) explains a significant proportion of the variance. The category of pre-eclampsia does not explain a significant proportion of the variance ($F = 0.42$) but its interaction with parity ($F = 3.14$, $p < 0.001$) and with smoking ($F = 2.35$, $p < 0.02$) are both significant although the interaction with sex of infant ($F = 0.56$) is not.

This analysis can be understood in relation to figure 11.2 which shows the mean corrected standardised birthweight scores by smoking and pre-eclampsia categories for the whole subsample of term babies.

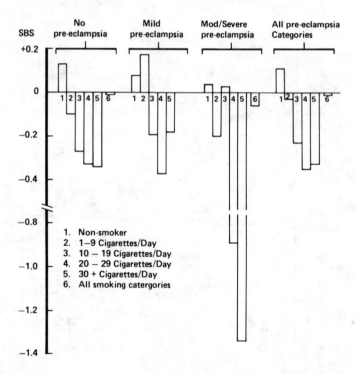

Figure 11.2   Mean corrected standardised birthweight scores by pre-eclampsia and smoking categories — term births

Overall, the differences in the classes of pre-eclampsia are not great although, with the exception of those who smoke between 10 and 19 cigarettes per day, the smallest standardised birthweight score in each smoking class is associated with proteinuric pre-eclampsia.

Figure 11.2 also indicates that the overall beneficial effect of hypertension without proteinuria has all but disappeared. The overall effect of proteinuric pre-eclampsia is reduced by the correction for maternal size, but among those women who smoke more than 20 cigarettes per day ($N = 17$), the effect of proteinuric pre-eclampsia is equally, if not more, marked. This might have been anticipated from the earlier observation (based on table 11.2) that these women tend to be heavy for their height, but any such prediction would have been foolhardy given the small numbers involved.

When the subsample is divided into groups according to sex of infant (table 11.4) the differences between the sexes by pre-eclampsia category are not great,

Table 11.4 Mean corrected standardised birthweight scores by pre-eclampsia and smoking categories and sex of infant — term births

Cigarettes per day	Pre-eclampsia							
	None mean	N	Mild mean	N	Prot. mean	N	All mean	N
(a) Boys								
0	0.13	1002	0.06	477	0.08	82	0.10	1561
−9	−0.15	94	0.18	40	−	−	−0.05	134
−19	−0.28	289	−0.20	98	0.05	14	−0.25	401
−29	−0.30	172	−0.25	66	−0.64	8	−0.30	246
30+	−0.24	30	−0.04	9	−1.18	2	−0.24	41
All	−0.02	1587	0.00	690	0.00	106	−0.01	383
(b) Girls								
0	0.14	913	0.11	429	−0.01	57	0.12	1399
−9	−0.04	82	0.14	31	−0.20	10	−0.01	123
−19	−0.25	257	−0.18	89	0.01	17	−0.22	363
−29	−0.35	184	−0.54	48	−1.22	6	−0.41	238
30+	−0.44	29	−0.26	15	−1.64	1	−0.42	45
All	−0.01	1465	0.01	612	−0.13	91	−0.01	2165

but are largest between the proteinuric groups. This difference is most marked between the proteinuric groups of those who smoke 20 cigarettes or more per day, which may be seen as part of a pattern of generally larger effects of heavier smoking on the birthweight of girls.

When the subsample is divided into parity groups (table 11.5) the overall effects of smoking are similar in each parity group. Amongst primiparae, the effects of pre-eclampsia are small, although there is a consistent positive effect of mild pre-eclampsia and a marked negative effect for the conjunction of proteinuric pre-eclampsia and smoking more than 19 cigarettes per day. For later born children mild pre-eclampsia has a detrimental effect, concentrated upon the group whose mothers smoked between 20 and 29 cigarettes per day. The effects of proteinuric pre-eclampsia are greater for later born than for first born children and are noticeable even among non-smokers. Smoking between 10 and 19

Table 11.5   Mean corrected standardised birthweight scores by pre-eclampsia smoking
categories and parity – term births

Cigarettes per day	Pre-eclampsia							
	None mean	N	Mild mean	N	Prot. mean	N	All mean	N
(a) Parity 0								
0	0.14	792	0.11	558	0.11	103	0.12	1453
–9	–0.07	88	0.27	46	–0.08	9	0.04	143
–19	–0.23	269	–0.24	120	–0.05	24	–0.22	413
–29	–0.37	149	–0.20	74	–0.77	9	–0.33	232
30+	–0.32	21	–0.13	16	–1.18	2	–0.29	39
All	–0.01	1319	0.03	814	0.00	147	0.00	2280
(b) Parity 1+								
0	0.13	1123	0.04	348	–0.14	36	0.10	1507
–9	–0.13	88	–0.02	25	–1.29	1	–0.12	114
–19	–0.30	277	–0.10	67	0.30	7	–0.25	351
–29	–0.29	207	–0.69	40	–1.10	5	–0.37	252
30+	–0.35	38	–0.27	8	–1.64	1	–0.36	47
All	–0.01	1733	–0.05	488	–0.22	50	–0.02	2271

cigarettes per day and proteinuric pre-eclampsia is, however, associated with a
higher than average corrected standardised birthweight score for later-born
children.

In general, then, the analysis of variance and the inspection of the mean
corrected standardised birthweight scores in cells defined by pre-eclampsia and
smoking categories suggest both that, among women who deliver later than 36
weeks gestation, the effects of pre-eclampsia are not great and that the previously
noted consistent effect of mild pre-eclampsia has all but disappeared. The effects
of proteinuric pre-eclampsia are, however, greater when the disorder occurs in
women bearing their second or subsequent child (cf. Campbell *et al.*, 1983a).
Moreover, the combination of smoking more than 19 cigarettes per day and
proteinuric pre-eclampsia seems particularly likely to lead to lower birthweight.

Corrections for maternal height among pre-term babies

The analysis is, again, constrained by the small numbers of pre-term births: there
are a total of 652 births with maternal height, smoking and pre-eclampsia data in
the sample. For the purposes of the ensuing analyses smoking categories above 9
cigarettes per day have been combined.

The analysis of variance shows that the main effects of smoking ($F = 9.82$,
$p < 0.001$) and pre-eclampsia ($F = 23.95, p < 0.001$) both account for significant proportions of the variance in the corrected standardised birthweight
scores. None of the interaction terms between either the variables at issue in this

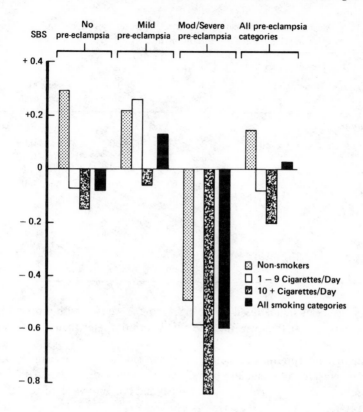

Figure 11.3   Mean corrected standardised birthweight scores by pre-eclampsia and smoking category — pre-term births

chapter or between them and those controlled for by the standardisation procedure is significant. Although detailed comparisons are not possible (because of small numbers), it is apparent that, while the effects of smoking dominated the analysis for term babies, for those born before 37 weeks gestation it is pre-eclampsia that accounts for the greatest proportion of the explained variance.

Figure 11.3 shows mean standardised birthweight scores for all pre-term births in smoking and pre-eclampsia categories. Overall, there is a positive effect of mild pre-eclampsia on the corrected standardised birthweight scores. The main difference between term and pre-term groups, however, is in the effects of proteinuric pre-eclampsia, where the mean standardised birthweight score is consistently less among pre-term than among term births.

When this sample is subdivided according to parity (table 11.6), the pattern of worse effects for proteinuric pre-eclampsia on the standardised birthweight score of later rather than first born, which was observed among term babies, is repeated for pre-term babies. For both primiparae and multiparae, however, the

Table 11.6   Mean corrected standardised birthweight scores by pre-eclampsia smoking
categories and parity – pre-term births

Cigarettes per day	Pre-eclampsia							
	None mean	N	Mild mean	N	Prot. mean	N	All mean	N
(a) Para 0								
0	0.19	102	0.24	36	−0.30	42	0.09	180
−9	−0.06	35	0.63	6	−0.54	13	−0.10	54
10+	−0.03	53	0.05	26	−0.53	17	−0.10	96
All	0.08	190	0.20	68	−0.40	72	0.00	330
(b) Para 1+								
0	0.37	120	0.20	27	−1.03	15	0.21	162
−9	−0.08	25	0.08	12	−1.05	1	−0.06	38
10+	−0.22	101	−0.23	17	−2.15	4	−0.28	122
All	0.08	246	0.04	56	−1.26	20	0.06	322

decrease in mean standardised birthweight score associated with proteinuric pre-eclampsia is greater than was the case for those born later than 36 weeks gestation.

Although interpreting such differences and similarities is hazardous because the numbers are so small, the overall pattern is not dissimilar to that noted among those whose pregnancy continued beyond the 36th week of gestation.

DISCUSSION

In general, the findings reported in this chapter correspond with those from other research. As early as 1957, Baird *et al.* reported from Aberdeen that:

> ...depression of birth...weight in pre-eclampsia is by no means general: a tendency to unusually low birth weights was found only in cases of severe pre-eclampsia in which delivery took place before term.

Similar findings have been noted by Long *et al.* (1980) and a more recent study by Moore and Redman (1983) has suggested that pre-eclampsia of early onset may differ from the late onset disease in aetiology and consequences.

With respect to maternal size, Butler and Alberman (1969) noted that severe pre-eclampsia was more commonly diagnosed in women of short stature, a finding also reported by Baird (1977). The issue of maternal weight is more contentious. Although the association between pre-eclampsia and obesity has been reported (e.g. Stewart and Hewitt, 1960), Lowe's (1961) findings suggest that obesity is not a significant risk factor in pre-eclampsia. While obesity as such has not been considered in the above analysis, it does appear that women who develop pre-eclampsia tend to be heavier for their height (table 11.2). The effect is particularly pronounced among women who are heavy smokers: indeed, the pattern of increases in mean z weights associated with increased cigarette consumption among those who develop mild and proteinuric pre-eclampsia is in marked contrast to the decrease in mean z weights associated with increased smoking among normotensive women.

The incidence of pre-eclampsia is significantly lower among those who smoke. This has also been noted by Butler and Alberman (1969) and others (e.g. Duffus and MacGillivray, 1968: Underwood *et al.*, 1965) have hypothesised that this might be related to the general hypotensive effects of smoking. The findings of this chapter indicate that mild pre-eclampsia offers some protection against the adverse effects of smoking. MacGillivray (1967) also noted the positive effects of mild pre-eclampsia on birthweight. In the more detailed analysis above, we have shown that this holds amongst *primiparae*, even when the effects of maternal weight are controlled, although smoking is still associated with decreased birthweight. Among *multiparae*, however, the effects of smoking more than 19 cigarettes per day and mild pre-eclampsia upon birthweight are similar to the effects of smoking at that level among normotensive women upon birthweight.

At several points in the analysis, we have noted that women who report smoking between 10 and 19 cigarettes per day are exceptions to the general patterns being noted. In particular, the adverse effects of proteinuric pre-eclampsia seem less severe for these women. This observation may correspond to the differential reporting effects hypothesised in the previous chapter.

Among primiparae who deliver later than 36 weeks, even proteinuric pre-eclampsia seems to afford some protection against the adverse effects of smoking less than 20 cigarettes per day. However, the joint effects of consumption of more than 19 cigarettes per day and proteinuric pre-eclampsia are greater than their additive effects. Both the independent effects of pre-eclampsia and the joint effects of pre-eclampsia and smoking on birthweight are greater for later than for first born babies whether they are born before or after 36 weeks gestation. The effects of pre-eclampsia are, however, greater among pre-term than among term babies and the joint negative effects of smoking and proteinuric pre-eclampsia are largest for later born pre-term babies whose mothers are heavy smokers.

Overall, our analysis indicates that for women who smoke more than 19 cigarettes per day, proteinuric pre-eclampsia is particularly likely to lead to lower birthweight babies and that heavy smokers who are above the average weight for their height are particularly prone to develop the disorder.

The analysis of this and the previous chapter cannot provide any definitive evidence reflecting on the debate about the causes of the association between smoking and reduced birthweight. Whilst the analysis of this and the previous chapter did show that increased cigarette consumption was associated with decreasing standardised birthweight scores, thereby suggesting a direct toxic effect, there is another interesting similarity between the two sets of results, the one controlling for social class and the other for the incidence of pre-eclampsia.

Thus, in chapter 10, we showed how among those who smoked 20 or more cigarettes per day, the positive effects of increasing maternal z weight upon standardised birthweight scores were significantly greater than among those who smoked less or who did not smoke. This finding would not be inconsistent with the suggestion that reduced calorific intake among smokers plays a part in the lower standardised birthweight score of their babies.

The analysis of this chapter suggests one possible mechanism for this effect. Women who are heavy for their height are more prone to develop mild pre-eclampsia which in turn is associated with a higher standardised birthweight score. However, we have also shown that independent of the effects of maternal weight-for-height, hypertension lessens the disadvantages of moderate maternal smoking to the baby. It is, therefore, possible that the antagonistic effects of maternal weight for height and smoking which we have observed arise because maternal weight for height confounds an antagonistic relation between maternal smoking and pre-eclampsia. Although, therefore, the analysis in this chapter does not refute a possible toxic effect of smoking, it does seem to provide some support for the hypothesis of nutritional differences between smokers and non-smokers.

SECTION 5

Summary and implications

12
Summary and implications for theory and practice

INTRODUCTION

Birthweight standards are important: they are used widely, both in the clinical assessment of the neonate and in epidemiological research. It is important, therefore, to understand them: the basis on which they have been and might be derived and how they relate to maternal characteristics and other features of the pregnancy. It is only in the light of this understanding that they can best be exploited whether for clinical or research purposes.

It became apparent to us that this would not be an easy task because of the difficulties we encountered when examining the trends in birthweight for gestation over the last thirty years within the unique data available at Aberdeen. The theoretical and statistical complexities in exploiting birthweight standards have been, in part, masked by the easy availability of look-up tables and nomograms. This monograph represents an attempt, as far as we are aware the first attempt, to examine the whole set of issues taking these complexities into account.

In particular, this monograph has shown how an explicit theoretical basis must be developed before statistical analysis can start; it is essential to have available good quality data and appropriate statistical methods; and the resulting standards demand care in their interpretation and use. This monograph has tried to use or provide all those things. The exercise has been relatively long (it is, after all, related to the analysis of but one set of data) and occasionally difficult. The argument has been that these difficulties are an inherent part of the subject and of the techniques required to tackle it. It is time, however, to summarise what has been learned and, in so doing, to point to areas of further research and make suggestions as to future research practice in this field.

The role of a couple of statisticians in making these kinds of suggestions may be questioned. It will be clear below — if it is not already obvious — that several issues are not dealt with at all: a good example is the whole question of heritability of size. However, the examination of the joint distribution of birthweight and gestation and the factors associated with it is quintessentially a statistical activity. Indeed, we would argue that the assessment of even an individual baby in the light of those distributions depends upon an understanding of them which, in turn, requires some statistical acumen. In consequence, we believe that the particular perspective afforded by careful theoretically based data analysis has a considerable amount to offer.

Partly because of the relative complexity of the statistical issues involved in developing birthweight standards, we have decided to provide a summary of the argument of the whole monograph, before considering the implications for methodology, substantive theory and the eventual use of standards. We realise that this entails a certain amount of repetition of material from previous chapters, but we think that this 'guided tour of the argument' will help set the context for the discussion that follows.

The main body of this chapter thereafter is divided into three sections. In the third section, we consider the implications of the methodological issues which have been confronted in the course of developing and exploiting the standards. Thus, we discuss the advantages of our model-building approach to the problem, the difficulties in the accurate measurement of gestation, our general strategy of avoiding statistical smoothing procedures, and the utility of the conventional division between pre-term and term. Then, in the fourth section, we consider the unresolved theoretical issues which have arisen as a result of our attempt to elaborate an overall model. Thus, we are still unclear as to what might be meant by a model of fetal growth, the role and status of non-normal factors has proved, whilst not intractable, problematic, and we have shown the importance of understanding the possible impact of variations in clinical practice. Finally, in the fifth section, we discuss the organisational and practical issues which arise when deriving and using the standards. Thus, on the one hand, we consider the quality and quantity of data required for estimating a set of birthweight standards, and on the other hand we draw attention to the ways in which they can be used, if used with care, whether in a clinical or research setting.

A GUIDED TOUR OF THE ARGUMENT

The background

The book started off by documenting the genesis of this study in the detailed comparison of recent birthweight surveys and in the puzzles provided by that comparison. One particular issue was highlighted: the relation between the pattern for birthweight-for-gestation and fetal growth. This leads on to the question of whether or not there is — or can be developed — a universally acceptable model of fetal growth. Taken together, these constitute a major theoretical problem confronted in this monograph.

At the same time, the introductory chapter draws out the importance of appreciating the uses to which the standards will be put. The clinical and research use of standards differ in their focus of concern (individual vs group); the factors used in defining standards (practicability vs research interest); form of standards (look-up tables vs statistically tractable); treatment of deviations from standards (management of pregnancy vs hypothesis testing); and the concept of 'normal' (hospital catchment area vs research problem). Whilst this monograph has emphasised the development and exploitation of research standards, many of the issues highlighted are also pertinent to the derivation and applicability of clinical standards.

Chapter 2 illustrates the puzzles which were provided by the comparison of birthweight surveys through an examination of the trends in birthweight for gestation over the last thirty years on the basis of the material available in the Aberdeen Maternity and Neonatal Data Bank. At first sight mean birthweight has hardly changed at all, the only shifts of any magnitude being a systematic decrease in the pre-term weeks. This pattern might be taken as support for Thomson's recent suggestion (1983) that already existing standards remain appropriate; with the decrease at pre-term weeks being taken as a consequence of well understood changes. However, our attempt to account for these decreases in terms of changes in induction practice, the relative proportion of primiparae and multiparae and the recorded incidence of pre-eclampsia led us to question the concept of normality represented by earlier standards. In turn, this suggested the need for a radical reappraisal of the basis of birthweight standards.

The theoretical argument

Chapters 3 and 4 constitute the knowledge base for the development of the theoretical model. The former chapter reviewed the evidence about the relationship between those factors which are assumed to affect fetal growth and observed birthweight. There have been controversies in the literature over the role of several factors. Three are of particular interest to this study: first, the appropriate method of parameterising maternal size in the examination of variations in birthweight, whether in terms of her height or weight; second, whether or not the mother's age does or does not have an independent effect upon birthweight; and third, what is the relation between higher parity and birthweight — some studies showing a continuing effect of parity whilst most have adopted the parsimonious dichotomy between first- and later-born. It is not pretended that the analysis of these issues provided later in the monograph offers a final resolution of them. In particular, we would suggest that the role of maternal age and multiparity can only be understood in the light of data on reproductive careers. However, we would also argue that, in the context of developing birthweight standards, the general approach adopted herein is the correct one, and that the particular solution which we have proposed to the problem is appropriate in the illustrative derivation of standards from the Aberdeen sample.

Chapter 4 is based on a review of a large number of birthweight surveys. We show that there has been a surprising diversity in the factors considered, the choice of base population and the sampling criteria for inclusion. The choice of factors to consider raises a whole set of issues about 'normality' and the relative importance of different kinds of factors. These are considered in the next chapter. Second, whilst the more usual hospital-based population potentially introduces biases and distortions, there are considerable advantages of uniformity in clinical practice and, importantly for retrospective analysis of this sort, in the collection and recording of data. Moreover, what would constitute a 'total population' on the basis of which distortion-free standards could be derived, is not obvious. Thirdly, no birthweight surveys can achieve complete coverage of a population, if only for technical reasons, and it is probably also sensible to systematically exclude cases of grave fetal malformation (e.g. anencephaly). But whatever the set of cases analysed, it is incumbent upon reports of birthweight surveys to be very specific about the criteria of selection they have used.

It is chapter 5 which sets this book apart from other birthweight surveys. The argument is developed that, without an explicit model of some kind, then it is not possible to provide an answer to controversies over, for example, the relative effect of maternal age and parity upon birthweight. Indeed, without some structure to guide inference, it is impossible to exploit the data other than to provide a statistical account of the variance of birthweight in a particular population. This was not the purpose of this study: indeed the overall explained variance is never reported.

The chapter sets out to model the process by which birthweight is determined. It demonstrates how the unknown degree of logical interdependence between fetal weight and the gestational age at onset of labour and the empirical difficulties encountered in making a precise estimate of gestational age independent of neonatal characteristics mean that the fetal growth process cannot be isolated or identified. This systematic ambiguity between the fetal growth process and observed distributions of birthweight is at the origin of several theoretical puzzles: for example, the consistently high standard deviation of birthweight at all gestational ages; and the difficulty of distinguishing between intrauterine growth retardation and prematurity.

Whilst a logically watertight model cannot therefore be developed, it is crucial, for the purposes of estimation, to impose at least a hierarchy upon the kinds of factors which can enter into a discussion of the determinants of variations in birthweight. On the basis of the attempt to develop a model, a hierarchical distinction is made between 'normal' and 'non-normal' factors. 'Normal' factors are taken as those which are present in every pregnancy and where the associated increment or decrement in the fetal growth rate does not of itself influence the prognosis for the baby. Fetal sex and gestational age at delivery are quintessentially 'normal' factors, whilst diseases of pregnancy such as maternal diabetes and pre-eclampsia are typical 'non-normal' factors. As with many categorisations it is not exhaustive: indeed, one of the advantages of the classification is that it focusses attention upon the relative status of 'intermediate' factors. 'Intermediate' factors are those which are present in every pregnancy but where the effects on growth rate may themselves influence prognosis or where the effects concerned may be confounded with the effects of non-normal factors. Of particular interest is the debate over the relative precedence of maternal height and weight, age and parity.

The empirical derivation of standards

Chapter 6 is the materials and methods chapter. The base population compares all live singleton births in the Aberdeen Maternity Hospital in 1975–1980. The hospital population provides larger numbers than a restricted geographical population and there were no obvious reasons for making such a restriction. Furthermore, it takes seriously the lessons which we draw from the review of other birthweight surveys that the quality of the data should be carefully examined and exclusions (and *a fortiori* inclusions) should be argued for. A particular issue in the Aberdeen population is the clinical practice of assigning an assessment of certainty both to information about the data of the last menstrual period and to the clinical estimate of gestation.

Chapters 7 and 8 set out to illustrate with the Aberdeen data the particular analytic strategy proposed as a consequence of the failure to derive an 'identifiable' system of equations. The preliminary analysis of the correlation matrix highlights the importance of knowing the local population and local clinical practice; another example is provided by the lack of association between maternal diabetes and birthweight which is almost certainly affected by the active monitoring and regulation of diabetes in Aberdeen. The first substantive step is to examine the intermediate factors with a view to making the analytic task more manageable. We decided at this stage of analysis to exclude maternal age and reduce the number of levels in parity.

The next issue dealt with in chapter 7 is the feasibility of fitting a functional form to the relationship between birthweight and gestation. On the one hand this would be very convenient — at least for clinical purposes. Whilst the logical interdependence between birthweight and gestation cannot, of course, be identified *via* such a curve-fitting exercise, it does provide some food for thought. A variety of functional forms are specified: the conclusion is that there are irreducible anomalies at 32, 37 and 42 weeks. We, therefore, argue that, even if convenience and clinical utility are the criteria, it is preferable to refer birthweights to an observed empirical distribution rather than a supposed fetal growth curve. Furthermore, the simplest theoretical explanation of the discrepancies is that the study population is a mixture of populations whose pregnancies follow different fetal curves.

Chapter 8 presents the basic standards: the means and standard deviations of birthweight in gestation/sex/parity cells. Birthweight scores, standardised to these distributions, are used in the remainder of the analyses. It is shown how it is possible to fit a statistical model for the effects of maternal weight and maternal weight-for-height without doing violence to the data. The analysis shows that there is a strong interaction between maternal height and weight-for-height and that the estimates based on a linear additive model are reduced for women who are short and light-for-their-height and tall and heavy-for-their-height; whilst they are increased for women who are short and heavy-for-their-height.

These standardised birthweight scores can, in this way, be corrected for the joint effects of maternal height and weight-for-height. Corrected standards are, in their turn, then used as a basis for the analysis of the residual effects of higher parity and of maternal age. In both cases, it is shown that the effects are probably spurious: higher parity selects for better reproducers; and age interacts with parity.

Applications to clinical and research contexts

In a sense, chapter 9 is a diversion from the main stream of the analysis in discussing clinical standards, but an important one. It shows how these standards, which were developed essentially for research use, can be easily translated into standards for clinical use. However, this translation highlights two problems — which might also affect the research use of standards. First, we demonstrate the extent to which the presumption of a normal distribution within gestation/ sex/parity cells could lead to misclassification. The alternative is to use the observed empirical distribution of birthweights within gestation/sex/parity cells and this raises the general problem of relying on the precise form of retrospective data in the assessment of future births (see below). Second, given the potential importance of the correction for maternal height and weight, the fact that there may be errors introduced by the assumption of constant parameters across gestations is an issue. It might be thought appropriate to standardise for birthweight within gestation/sex/parity/maternal height/maternal weight cells: but this raises the problem of finding sufficient cases from a homogeneous population. We conclude by emphasising that our view as statisticians is that standards should be used as an *aid* to clinical judgement and not as a clinical assessment in their own right.

Chapters 10 and 11 are illustrative of the way in which standards can be used to address research questions. Substantively, they raise questions about the complex association of smoking and birthweight in the light of the effects of social class, maternal size and pre-eclampsia. In particular, chapter 10 shows how the effects of social class on mean birthweight can be accounted for either by maternal size or by smoking habits. However, continuing detrimental effects of lower social class within the distributions of standardised birthweight scores are noted. Chapter 11 shows how the effects of smoking, maternal size and pre-eclampsia are in some cases counteracting and in others reinforcing. In both cases the association between the effects of maternal size and smoking habits provides support for a hypothesis that nutritional differences play some part in the observed deleterious effects of smoking.

These chapters also have a more general lesson in that they show that the 'non-normal' factors within a sample affect the relationships between 'normal' and 'intermediate' factors and birthweight: a point that is further discussed below.

IMPLICATIONS FOR METHODOLOGY

In some ways the major lessons from our work are methodological. Thus it is important: to stress the considerable efforts to which we went to develop a model prior to the derivation of standards of birthweight; to underline both the practical and theoretical difficulties of measuring 'true' gestation; to emphasise an approach to analysis which remains close to the data; and to be particularly careful in using the conventional divisions between pre-term and term.

Why a model?

Our emphasis on building a model can be simply explained. First, we would claim that any kind of analysis of birthweight distributions contains an *implicit* model with its attendant assumptions and presumptions. In exploring the consequences of these hidden assumptions and presumptions, it is essential to set forth an *explicit* model. At the same time, we would argue that, in this field, where a considerable amount of research knowledge is available on each of the issues involved, there is no excuse for the kind of exploratory data analysis which may seem appropriate in more uncharted fields. Instead, we must incorporate existing knowledge into a specification of a structural model which imposes, as far as is possible, a causal ordering among the variables in the analysis. This structure is then used to test hypotheses about these interrelationships at the same time as searching for a best fit solution for the model.

Even where, as proved to be the case here, it is impossible to specify a *complete* model, it would *not* be appropriate to ignore what is known and simply to look for an equation with maximum predictive power. Thus, one could *predict* likely birthweight very well using maternal weight near term or, even better, the gain in maternal weight over the pregnancy. But, whilst the study of the rate of maternal weight gain at each week of the pregnancy might eventually help to illuminate (together with the study of other changes) the fetal growth process, it would not provide sensible or usable standards for the resulting birthweight. The fact that there is a strong association between the gain in maternal weight and achieved fetal weight tells us nothing about what is, or what is not, normal, or how to identify growth retarded babies. Indeed, we want to stress that the objective of the exercise is *not* to *account for* as much of the variance in birthweight as possible in terms of other factors: thus we never report the explained variance.

Instead, the objective of a birthweight survey should be to distinguish between the kinds of factors which affect birthweight and to quantify their relative influence. To do this, it proved essential to incorporate existing knowledge into the specification of a baseline model – even if it is only a partial one. For example, the treatment of high multiparity and maternal age required a particular framework within which the effects could be evaluated. Furthermore, it is only through a specified model that we can look for non-linearities – such as the interaction between maternal height and weight – which have been a major feature of the development of the standards for research use. Without a model framework, there would have been no reason to explore those interactions in preference to any others.

Whilst the solutions we have adopted and the answers we have obtained are specific to this particular data set, we claim that any examination of the relationship between birthweight and other factors would benefit from setting forth an explicit model before analysis starts.

Measurement of length of gestation

The 'true' length of gestation is the interval between fertilisation and the date of delivery. For practical reasons, however, the almost universal method of calculating gestation is to subtract the day of the Last Menstrual Period from the date of delivery and record this in numbers of completed weeks. The approximation introduced by this particular rounding procedure – which on its own introduces a possible error of up to six days – is compounded by doubts about the relation of the date of menstruation to the dates of ovulation and fertilisation. The review of the evidence in chapter 3 suggests that this latter difference may vary by as much as a week from the presumed fourteen days. At best, therefore, a recorded gestation (based on perfectly accurate information about the last menstrual period) of 39 completed weeks could actually refer to a length of gestation between 266 days (38 completed weeks) and 286 days (one day less than 41 completed weeks). If further, we acknowledge the possibility that the pregnant mother is uncertain or ambiguous about her dates, then the potential range of, say, a nominal 39 week gestation is enormous.

It is clearly unsatisfactory that at least potentially there should be such large discrepancies between the 'true' length of gestation and the values actually recorded for the gestation variable – which accounts for by far the largest proportion of the variation in birthweight. It is true that one part of the errors in measurement, that which arises from cases where there are uncertainties over the dates of the Last Menstrual Period, can, in principle, be avoided by excluding such cases from the analysis. It should be noted, however, that if an external criterion – such as ultrasound measurement – is used, then this presumes that the criterion were validated on perfect dates (vide Hall *et al.*,

1984). The approach adopted in this study has been to restrict the analysis to cases where the gestation has been assessed by the clinical staff. Whilst this avoids that particular presumption about validation, the problem posed by doubts about the relation between the date of menstruation and the dates of ovulation and fertilisation remain.

It is clearly impracticable to envisage a birthweight survey where every case has been monitored since conception with sufficient numbers. Users of birthweight standards must, therefore, be aware of the (relatively large) potential range of 21 days in the gestation variable. Whilst on the whole this is simply a nuisance in the research use of standards (but see the section on the Role and Status of Non-normal Factors below) in the clinical context, it is important to realise that the assessment of 'light-for-dates' or 'heavy-for-dates' depends upon the unverifiable presumption that the recorded number of completed weeks exactly reflects the 'true' length of gestation.

These practical problems of measuring the length of gestation are compounded, in the analysis of variations in birthweight, by the logical *inter*dependence between the length of gestation and achieved fetal growth. For not only does birthweight depend on the length of gestation and the onset of labour but, therefore, the length of gestation may well depend on achieved fetal growth. As we explained in chapter 5, this means that we cannot estimate the structural parameters of the system but only the coefficients of the single equation model where birthweight is the dependent variable being affected by gestation (and the other factors) ignoring the possible dependence of gestation upon birthweight. In turn, this means that the estimated coefficients cannot be taken as reflecting the parameters of a fetal growth process (see below).

The empirical approach

It may seem curious that, with all this computational power available, we have developed rather old-fashioned birthweight standards. Recent workers have estimated a functional relation between birthweight and gestation (e.g. Altman and Coles, 1980); others have proposed a variety of smoothing procedures (e.g. Thomson *et al.*, 1968). Whilst convenient, the presumption (in both cases) is that there is a unique process of fetal growth which can be approximated by the observed joint distribution of birthweight and gestation. We have argued strongly against this view and suggested that it is far more plausible to suppose that the observed distributions are an outcome of a particular but unknowable mix of several fetal growth processes.

We do not, therefore, make any presumption about the pattern of fetal growth and, in particular, we do not presume that there is one functional relation between birthweight and gestation to be estimated on the basis of the observed distributions. Instead, we advocate the initial standardisation of birthweights to the empirical distributions within gestation/sex/parity cells. Whilst this may appear cumbersome, it has the considerable advantage of remaining close to the data. Note that this implies that applicability of standards developed in one particular place at one particular time in any other context cannot be assumed: whether or not they are applicable should always be checked empirically. Indeed, even within the same population, the use of standardised birthweight scores assumes that there are equivalent distributions of birthweights across the 44 gestation/sex/parity cells. The typical presumption of normality only makes matters worse.

It is true that we have been forced to compromise this thoroughly empirical approach in the development of the correction for maternal height and weight. In principle, this inconsistency could be overcome with a very large amount of data so that one could standardise birthweights to the distribution within a gestation/sex/parity/maternal height/maternal weight cell. On the whole, we think that would be unrealistic. For, in order to obtain sufficient cases, the data would have to be collected over a large number of hospitals (or areas), or over a long period of time. In both cases, the advantages of uniformity both of clinical practice and of the collection and recording of data, when the data is collected from one hospital (or area) over a relatively short-time period, would be lost.

We, therefore, suggest that corrections of maternal size should be calculated by some statistical method of the kind employed in chapter 8. As far as it goes, that is unproblematic: the trouble comes as soon as we start to use these corrected standardised birthweight scores as a means of comparing birthweights across gestation/sex/parity cells. (The problem has already been considered in respect of the *un*corrected standardised birthweight scores). For, whilst the analysis showed that it was statistically appropriate to assume constant coefficients across the gestational ages, the estimated correction for an *individual* baby born, for example, at 32 weeks, may not be. Once again, the conclusion is that whether or not a set of standards is applicable to a specific population is a problem which requires empirical verification.

The boundary between pre-term and term

The division into pre-term and term at 36/37 weeks is, of course, acknowledged to be conventional and, to that extent, it is arbitrary. Thus, the attempt at curve-fitting and relation between birthweight and gestation in chapter 7 was unsatisfactory, partly because it was found that a better fit could be obtained by splitting the population at 37/38 (rather than 36/37) weeks. Even if this finding were to be replicated elsewhere, this does not mean that the definition of pre-term should be changed — it is, after all, a useful convention providing a common language for the discussion of intrauterine growth retardation, among other things. It does, nevertheless, mean that research about the differences between pre-term and term should pay particular attention to possible overlaps at 36 and 37 weeks.

Indeed, it is worth noting that different definitions-in-practice are used. Thus, Bakketeig and Hoffman (1979), in their large scale longitudinal study, use the division 35/36 weeks. In this study we were struck by the fact that the difference in birthweight between those induced and those not induced occurs at or before 35 weeks and not at all thereafter. This was interpreted as reflecting the active management of pre-term pregnancies — but, in this case, 'pre-term' seems to stop at 35 (rather than 36) weeks.

In deriving birthweight standards, the arbitrariness of the division implies that it is always an open question as to where the division between 'pre-term' and 'term' should be located. Indeed, whether or not the data from the separate gestational weeks can be combined for the purposes of estimating coefficients is an empirical question (see below).

IMPLICATIONS FOR RESEARCH

It is incumbent upon academics to participate in a collective job-creation exercise by proposing further research. Yet, cynicism apart, there are three sets of issues which have been raised by this analysis: deeper understanding of the process of fetal growth, the role and status of 'non-normal' factors, and the likely effects of clinical practice upon birthweight distributions.

Research on fetal growth

The model development in chapter 5 attempted to bring together what was known about the process of fetal growth and its relation to observed birthweight into one model structure. Nevertheless, it has to be acknowledged that three issues were treated rather summarily.

First, the specification of the model came unstuck in attempting to incorporate the possible dependence of gestational age at delivery upon fetal weight. That argument, of course, relates to deliveries following spontaneous onset of labour: it seems obvious that the more active the management of pregnancy, the less gestational age at delivery will depend upon fetal weight. Yet, whilst the analysis in chapter 2 did show a dramatic difference between the birthweights of those induced and those not induced among babies born at 35 weeks or earlier, there was no discernible difference among later deliveries (see also chapter 7). Spontaneous onset of labour is clearly different from induced labour: the question is how does that difference relate to the fetal growth rate?

At the same time, the consistently high standard deviations of birthweight even when standardised within gestation/sex/parity cells is a puzzle. The prevalence of induction at pre-term weeks in this population and the fact that those babies who are induced pre-term are about 250 g lighter possibly provides a small part of the answer. But the finding of a high standard deviation is not unique to this population. Instead, we would suggest that a major reason is the inaccuracy with which the length of gestation is inevitably measured. Thus, a nominal gestation group of, say, 35 weeks, contains an unknown mix of 'true' gestation lengths of 34, 35 and 36 weeks (and even some of 37 weeks — see the section on The Measurement of the Length of Gestation (above)). Whilst, however, this would have a substantial effect on the distribution of birthweights in a pre-term nominal gestation group such as this — of the order of 200 g either way — this would still not account for the equally high standard deviation in the term nominal gestation groups.

We have, however, argued that another possible explanation is that the observed distribution of birthweight for gestation is the consequence of a mixture of distributions corresponding to different processes of fetal growth. To advance understanding it would, therefore, be crucial to identify the subpopulations who are relatively homogeneous in respect of their process of fetal growth. Given the apparent inability to reduce the variance in birthweight substantially, despite considerable research endeavour, it would seem worthwhile to search for a subpopulation which is relatively homogeneous in respect of their pattern of fetal growth (cf. Naeye and Dixon, 1978). Instead of attempting to identify an 'ideal' fetal growth curve, the focus of research would be on the investigation of the distinctive characteristics of these 'homogeneous' groups. groups.

Second, the whole question of the effect of the woman's previous obstetric history upon birthweight was avoided. Whilst information on previous spontaneous abortions and induced terminations is collected, and could have been incorporated in the statistical analysis, it is argued that this kind of question is best answered *via* career-wise analysis. The effect upon the model is also unclear: a record of previous spontaneous abortions would perhaps indicate a poor reproducer — that is, someone whose pregnancies will, *even if they continue to term*, follow a different path than others; but it may also result from a specific disease or illness during pregnancy.

Whatever the reason, subgroups of mothers do follow different paths of fetal growth. This can be illustrated as follows. The difference between births at 35 and 36 weeks corresponds to a difference in birthweights of 211.4 g (para 0 boys): this reflects not only 1 week's growth *in utero* but also a decrease in the proportion of proteinuric eclamptics (from 28.9% to 12.7%) and an increase in mild pre-eclamptics (from 13.3% to 22.8%), and many other changes in the distribution of other non-normal factors which we do not know about.

Third, there is the whole question of the relative balance between genetic and environmental factors. For example, although it has proved possible to tease out the covariation of standards with maternal height and weight-for-height, this was on the (reasonable) assumption that adult height should take precedence over maternal weight in modelling the variations in birthweight. On the other hand, adult height clearly depends upon nutrition in childhood: in most statistical models this would be measured by adolescent weight which is, of course, strongly predictive of adult weight.

The basic problem is that this kind of question cannot be answered by a birthweight survey of this type. Whilst some clues can be obtained by exploring the relation between the birthweights of different sets of relatives, that kind of research has regrettably been relatively scarce over the last twenty years. But the original question can only be properly answered with a longitudinal study collecting detailed information on (the factors affecting) physical development during childhood and adolescence and adult reproductive performance.

The role and status of 'non-normal' factors

This book has argued for the importance of distinguishing between 'normal', 'intermediate' and 'non-normal' factors, and for standardising for both 'normal' and 'intermediate' factors before investigating the effects of 'non-normal' factors. Clearly, there are a multitude of 'non-normal' factors whose effects could be investigated: the particular topics chosen for inclusion in this monograph are but two examples.

The topics chosen are also exemplary in that we can draw general lessons from them. Thus, the detailed analysis in those chapters showed that, whilst it would be convenient to ignore the role of factors which have been incorporated into the standards, life is not so simple. In fact, the analysis in those chapters turned in one case upon the specific distribution of maternal weight in cells defined by the cross-classification of smoking habits and social class, and in the other, upon the bizarre distributions of pre-eclampsia and smoking habits within the maternal height and maternal weight-for-height distributions.

Another issue that was avoided in both chapters was the 'validity' of the categories being used. Thus, the fact that the effects of social class can be accounted for by the effects of smoking and/or maternal weight-for-height poses as many questions as it answers. As has been suggested elsewhere (see Illsley and Mitchell, 1984) the social class classification is a particularly crude instrument for capturing the effect of the environment upon pregnancy. A related point can be made about both pre-eclampsia and smoking habits, which are socially constructed categories; the first, since the definitions of pre-eclampsia are by no means universal; the second, since the recording of smoking habits depends on self-reported data and there is good evidence to suggest that honesty is socially differentiated (see below).

On the one hand, therefore, future research into the effects of 'non-normal' factors upon birthweight scores should take great care over the possible interactions between different levels of that factor and the factors incorporated into the birthweight scores. At the same time, there is also a place for research into the joint distribution of these particular 'non-normal' factors with 'normal' factors among the 'at risk' population, paying particular attention to the quality of the data.

Research on the importance of local clinical practice

At two points in the book, the analysis has turned upon local clinical practice.

For example, the basic standards population includes only those cases where the clinical estimate of gestation has been assessed as certain because of the problems of simultaneity discussed in chapter 5. This entailed the exclusion of nearly one quarter of the population (see chapter 6 and its Data Appendix). The study of the distribution of birthweight among women whose gestations have been assessed as uncertain would clearly pay dividends. But not on this population – there are not enough data (see below).

Similarly, the analysis in chapter 2 highlighted the different distributions of birthweights among those induced and those not induced pre-term. The extent to which further research here would pay dividends in terms of understanding the onset of spontaneous labour has already been mentioned. But there is also the question of induction itself. Quite apart from the interests of clinical audit, there remains the problem of the extent to which induction identifies a group or groups where the mother or the fetus was 'at risk'. The consequences in terms of the distribution of birthweight for gestation have been discussed but, in addition, the identification of such 'at risk' groups may result in different relationships between birthweight for gestation and the prognosis for the baby in such groups. In circumstances where 40 per cent of labours are induced, such a suggestion would have important implications for both birthweight standards and for obstetric epidemiology.

There are other instances of changes in clinical practice which could usefully be explored. Thus, the changing rate of induced abortions (Pritchard and Thompson, 1982) may well have implications for the birthweight distributions: both because of the possible overlaps with what would otherwise be cases of intrauterine growth retardation and because there might be career-wise relations between an abortion (spontaneous or induced) and preceding or subsequent births. Moreover, clinical practice may, of itself, change the distributions of a 'non-normal' factor thereby rendering analysis more complex. For example, the concept of 'gestational diabetes' was new with Lund and Weese's (1953) seminal paper and it may be that in future Sutherland *et al.*'s (1970) suggestion of wider screening for gestational diabetes will change the whole conception of the distribution of the 'non-normal' factor of abnormal glucose tolerance.

The problem of excluded groups

In the process of developing standards of birthweight for gestation, we have excluded three groups from discussion.

By far the largest such group arose because of our decision to exclude those cases where the length of gestation could not be determined reliably by the clinical staff – what in Aberdeen are referred to as 'uncertain' or 'approximate' gestations. This group accounted for some 23% of *all* singleton live births at the Aberdeen Maternity Hospital during this period. We excluded them because, in the end, it is obviously absurd to produce *standards* of birthweight-for-gestation when you cannot have *any* confidence in the raw data for the length of gestation.

In the Aberdeen context, we were fortunate that there has been a concerted effort on the part of the clinicians to assess the certainty of gestation in every case; and we would recommend that where standards of birthweight-for-gestation are to be developed, there should be a routine check on the quality of the basic gestation data.

Clearly, there are contexts where it is impossible in the majority of cases for a clinician, and *a fortiori* a researcher, to be confident about the length of gestation with any accuracy in this way, for example where there is limited or no ante-natal care. The suggestion that, in such cases, we might use birthweight standards developed elsewhere does not help: for the variation in the estimates of gestation may well be related to variations in the outcome and the argument in chapters 5 and 9 implies that the utility of any set of standards depends on the local conditions. As a corollary, it would be absurd to use standards of birthweight-for-gestation as a basis for estimating the length of gestation given the achieved birthweight.

In such contexts, there are probably many more urgent matters to worry about than the development of birthweight standards, but if assessment of birthweight were thought important, the research objective would be to look for another method of assessing the length of gestation. The promise of ultra-sound scanning is illusory: for the technology will not, usually in such cases, be routinely available; moreover standards of fetal growth derived from ultrasound measurements still depend, ultimately, on the assumption of perfect dates for the sample on which they were validated.

There were two other groups of exclusions: stillbirths and twins (or triplets, etc.). The former, which accounted for rather less than 1% of all singleton births at Aberdeen Maternity Hospital, were excluded because, in the majority of cases, we cannot be certain as to the length of gestation. Indeed, we would claim that birthweight standards have nothing to offer in the case of macerated stillbirths – when both gestation and weight at death are uncertain. These accounted for the majority of stillbirths in Aberdeen. In other cases it might be appropriate to refer the birthweight to locally developed standards as an aid to the differential diagnosis of cause of death, but only where the time of death *is* known.

Multiple births, which accounted for about one in eighty of all maternities at Aberdeen Maternity Hospital pose more of a problem. Whilst not represent-ing a large number of births, given the greatly increased perinatal risk, it would clearly be useful if birthweight standards could assist in the assessment of fetal growth. But, it seems very unlikely that there would ever be sufficient numbers of multiple births for the derivation of clinically useful local standards to be feasible. For research purposes, standards of birthweight-for-gestation (of a sort) could possibly be derived for a large population ignoring the constraints of locality. There remains a fundamental problem: it is unclear whether the relative lightness of a twin should be interpreted with reference to singleton standards – in which case nearly all twins are 'light-for-dates' – or whether this relative lightness results from a 'normal' pattern of fetal growth *sui generis*. Clearly a wide range of research issues are involved.

DERIVING AND USING STANDARDS IN A PARTICULAR SETTING

This monograph has focussed on the epidemiological analysis of the distribution of birthweight in a particular sample. It has, however, led us to make a series of recommendations for those who would like to use birthweight standards in a research setting, both in terms of the quality and quantity of data that should be collected, and the general strategy that should be adopted to their derivation. We go on to make some tentative suggestions as to the regular monitoring of trends in birthweight-for-gestation, and the use of appropriate standards by the clinician both in considering an individual case and as an alternative to a case-control design.

Quality of data

The authors have been very fortunate in this study in terms of the quality of the data that has been routinely recorded at the Aberdeen Maternity Hospital: others may not be so lucky. Nevertheless, there are two variables for which it might be helpful either to routinely collect extra data, or where coding practices need clarification.

Thus, data on smoking habits is in the majority of studies self-reported. It is known that self-reporting of certain events and incidents such as own delinquency and victimisation by others (OECD, 1976) varies according to social class. The same is quite likely to be true of smoking habits in that middle-class women may be more likely to know that they 'ought' not to be smoking and to reduce either consciously or unconsciously the number they report.

Problems with the measurement of gestation have been mentioned several times in this chapter. In order to estimate even the reduced form of the model developed in chapter 5, cases of uncertain gestation had to be excluded. This was not because of the increased range *per se* although one would probably want to exclude uncertain gestations in any case — because of the large possible error (± 4 weeks) implied by that assessment. The fundamental problem is that the assessment of uncertain (or approximate) gestations implies that there had been a conflict between some of the evidence available — and some of this evidence might relate to neonatal characteristics. The only sure way to avoid this problem is to restrict the analysis to cases where the mother is certain about the date of her last menstrual period and has a regular menstrual cycle. This is effectively what is meant by our restriction to certain gestations.

Quantity of data

It seems curious for a brace of data analysts to be complaining about lack of data having just number-crunched their way through some 17 000 cases. But the complaint is real enough if one wants to investigate seriously the influence of certain – possibly most – 'non-normal' factors. For example, part of the argument in chapter 10 turned on the values for 17 cases. *Extremely* large samples are, in some cases, necessary to do justice to an analysis.

On the other hand, the 'weights' sample used to illustrate the derivation of standards had less than 5000 cases. Nonetheless, it has proved possible to derive standardised birthweight scores for this sample which were very similar to the scores for those babies when the standardised birthweight scores were calculated for the whole 'standards' sample.

Thus, although certain avenues of research are restricted by small numbers, this should not be seen as an impediment to the derivation of the basic standardised birthweight scores in the context of a medium-sized hospital population.

The general strategy

We have, on several occasions, advocated the derivation of locally based standards. Indeed, one of the intentions in going through the procedure of deriving standards has been to demonstrate a general strategy. However, this falls short of providing some sort of universal recipe. The *actual content* of the various stages of the procedure must depend on the particular circumstances pertaining at a particular time and place and on the results of the preceding stage of analysis. On the other hand, although we are unwilling to recommend a universal technique, the analyses presented in this book do suggest that the calculation of standardised birthweight scores for gestation/sex/parity cells provides an easy way of deriving standards which avoids many of the analytic difficulties.

Corrections for maternal conformation, however, pose considerably more problems. Whilst we would, in general, recommend the step-by-step approach followed in chapter 8, it cannot be presumed, in another context, that a set of uniform coefficients will actually correspond to the joint distributions of maternal height and weight with birthweight-for-gestation, as they did in our case. In particular, we were lucky in that, whilst a uniform coefficient for maternal weight over all gestational ages was not appropriate, there appeared to be a convenient break between 36 and 37 weeks, which, of course, corresponds to the conventional division between pre-term and term.

However, although the appropriateness of a linear model cannot be presumed, a sensible first attempt would be to estimate the regression of the basic standardised birthweight scores on maternal height, maternal weight and their interaction (perhaps separately for pre-term and term). These coefficients could then be used to calculate a set of corrections for maternal size within the larger maternal height/maternal weight cells. If this set of corrections are predictively accurate, then these same coefficients could probably safely be used throughout the range. Otherwise the appropriateness of any coefficient across two or more gestation/sex/parity cells must be checked empirically as in chapter 8.

The regular monitoring of birthweight

There are two 'organisational' implications arising from the argument for the desirability of developing and using current locally based standards.

The first is that standards quickly get out-of-date. In Aberdeen, there had apparently been little change in mean birthweight over a quarter of a century, but the closer scrutiny in chapter 2 showed that there had been fundamental shifts in the nature of the birthweight distribution, especially at the pre-term weeks. In consequence, we restricted our sample to a recent seven-year period.

In general, we would recommend the frequent checking of the distributions, not only of birthweight-for-gestation but also of the other factors associated with birthweight. Indeed, where resources are available, we would advocate the repeated derivation of birthweight standards (say, annually) on the basis of a rolling five-year reference period. Similarly, this process of monitoring will provide valuable information for a clinical audit.

Such an ambitious programme would, of course, call upon the skills of an in-house statistician. Whilst this could be viewed as another instance of special pleading, the more serious point is that in order that for any set of standards to be used appropriately, a level of statistical acumen is crucial.

The clinical use of standards

The question of the utility of birthweight standards has been raised at several points in the monograph. The concluding discussion of chapter 9 counselled caution in the clinical use of standards. They — whether the home-grown empirical variety advocated here or nomograms based on a smoothing procedure and an assumption of normality — should be used as an *aid* to, but not as a substitute for, the clinical assessment of individual babies.

However, although we have been unable to offer comfortable reassurance to the clinician, birthweight standards remain one of the best ways available of answering the question of whether a baby's size is appropriate to its gestational age. As such they should properly continue to play their part in paediatric assessment. Our words of caution have been directed towards the over-rigid use of statistical diagnostic criteria especially in the pre-term weeks. On the other hand, for research use in a clinical context, birthweight standards derived in the way described may have considerable utility. For, since the standards control for several factors at once, they permit the study of birthweight as an outcome in studies where there are relatively few cases without recourse to the exigencies of case control. In the same way, if locally based standards are available, experimental designs or studies of comparatively rare complications of pregnancy (such as maternal diabetes) become easier to carry out.

However, problems may arise in their use because of the particular distribution of non-normal factors in the population. Thus, one might want to use standards so as to monitor the success of antenatal care, growth retardation and, in particular, to determine the appropriateness of pre-term induction practices. Taking the standards developed in this monograph as an example, one must be aware that they were derived from a sample in which 21.8% of pre-term births were to mothers with proteinuric pre-eclampsia of which over three-quarters (76.1%) were induced. The standard of 'normal' weight for dates thus incorporated a substantial proportion of babies who may have significantly depressed fetal growth, and monitoring using categories derived from the standards may systematically underestimate the proportions affected.

CONCLUDING REMARKS

The analysis in this study has a specific focus: the development of birthweight standards via an empirical and statistical model for the Aberdeen population in recent years. But this analysis is intended as an illustration of an overall strategy, in particular the general approach advocated in chapter 5 and chapters 7-11.

We make no apology for saying again that analyses of this kind *always* require the development of a formal model as a basis for estimation: in fact, very few birthweight surveys even address the conceptual issues raised in chapter 5 on the basis of the discussion in chapters 3 and 4. Even where – as in this case – the full structural model cannot be estimated, then some *a priori* structuring of the factors is required if the analysis is to provide anything more than a statistical account of the variance in birthweight. In chapter 5 we advocated a distinction between 'normal' and 'non-normal' factors: whether or not this is universally accepted, some such distinction is required.

In chapters 7-11 we have shown how the specific content of the standards depends upon the particular empirical distributions which obtain in the data. Indeed, the message of all the analyses in chapters 7-11 is that standards of birthweight for gestation which are *specific* both in location and time should be developed wherever there is enough data. On the other hand, we think that the *general* strategy for deriving standards can be applied wherever there is sufficient good quality data.

Indeed, we claim that the development of such locally based standards would have a number of advantages. First, they would be appropriate in the context of the particular local distribution of 'normal' and 'non-normal' factors and in ensuring relative uniformity of clinical practice and the collection and recording of data. Second, in contrast to our earlier caveats about the direct clinical applications of standards, we believe that the clinician could correctly place more reliance in locally based standards. For these kinds of reasons we would strongly advocate the development of standards on the basis of any medium sized hospital population.

Finally, the arguments in this book should urge caution on all those who would use the observed distributions of birthweight as a guide to understanding processes of fetal growth. Indeed, much of the further research proposed in this chapter is oriented towards profitting from birthweight distributions in specific subpopulations as an aid to that understanding. Above all, what this study has demonstrated, we believe, is that much can be learnt in this field, from the development and testing of a formal model.

References

Adams, M. S. and Niswander, J. D. (1968). Birthweight of North American Indians, *Human Biol.*, **40**, 226–34

Adamson, K. and Joelsson, I. (1977). The effects of pharmacologic agents upon the fetus and newborn. In: *Current Developments in Perinatology: the Fetus, Placenta and Newborn* (ed. F. P. Zuopan), C. V. Mosby & Co., St Louis, pp. 531–54

Altman, D. G. and Coles, E. C. (1980). Assessing birthweight-for-dates on a continuous scale, *Ann. Hum. Biol.*, **7** (1), 35–44

Andrews, J. and McGary, J. M. (1972). A community study of smoking in pregnancy, *J. Obs. Gynaec. Br. Commonw.*, **79**, 1057

Antonov, A. N. (1947). Children born during the siege of Leningrad in 1942, *J. Paediatr.*, **30**, 250–59

Baird, D. (1977). Epidemiological aspects of hypertensive pregnancy, *Clin. Obstet. Gynaecol.*, **4**, 531–48

Baird, D., Thomson, A. M. and Billewicz, W. Z. (1957). Birthweights and placental weights in pre-eclampsia, *J. Obstet. Gynaecol. Br. Emp.*, **64**, 370–72

Bakketeig, L. S. and Hoffman, J. H. (1979). Perinatal mortality by birth order within cohorts based on sibships size, *Br. med. J.*, **ii**, 693–96

Barron, S. L. (1983). Birthweight and ethnicity, *Br. J. Obstet. Gynaec.*, **90**, 289–90

Barron, S. L. and Vessey, M. P. (1966). Birthweight of infants born to immigrant mothers, *Br. J. prev. soc. Med.*, **20**, 127–34

Batson, G. A. (1974). Cyanotic congenital heart disease in pregnancy, *J. Obstet. Gynaec. Br. Commonw.*, **81**, 549–53

Battaglia, F. C., Frazier, T. M. and Hellegers, A. E. (1966). Birthweight, gestational age and pregnancy outcome, with special reference to the high birthweight low gestational age infant, *Pediatrics*, **37**, 417–22

Billewicz, W. Z., Kemsley, W. F. F. and Thomson, A. M. (1962). Indices of adiposity, *Br. J. prev. soc. Med.*, **16**, 183–88

Billewicz, W. Z. and Thomson, A. M. (1973). Birthweights in consecutive pregnancies, *J. Obstet. Gynaec. Br. Commonw.*, **80**, 491–98

Birkbeck, J. A. Billewicz, W. Z. and Thomson, A. M. (1975). Human fetal measurements between 50 and 150 days of gestation, *Ann. Hum. Biol.*, **2**, 319–26

Bishop, E. H. (1964). Maternal heart volume and prematurity, *JAMA*, **187**, 500–2

Blinick, G., Walloch, R. C., Jerez, E. and Ackerman, B. D. (1976). Drug addiction in pregnancy and the neonate, *Am. J. Obstet. Gynec.*, **125**. 135–41

Bolton, R. N. (1959). Some considerations of excessive fetal development: a study of 144 cases, *Am. J. Obstet. Gynec.*, 77, 118-27

Brenner, W. E., Edelman, D. A. and Hendricks, C. M. (1976). A standard of fetal growth for the United States of America, *J. Obstet. Gynec.*, 126, 555-64

Brent, R. Z. and Jensch, R. P. (1967). Intrauterine growth retardation, *Adv. Teratol.*, 2, 139-227

Butler, N. L. and Alberman, E. D. (1969). *Perinatal Problems*, Livingstone, Edinburgh

Camilleri, A. P. and Cremona, V. (1970). The effect of parity on birthweight, *J. Obstet. Gynaec. Br. Commonw.*, 77, 145-47

Campbell, D. M., Carr-Hill, R. and Orisaseyi, A. E. (1983a). Pre-eclampsia in a second pregnancy, *Clin. Exper. Hyper. Pregn.*, B2 (2), 303-6

Campbell, D. M. and MacGillivray, I. (1975). The effects of a low calorie diet on a thiazide diuretic on the incidence of pre-eclampsia and on birthweight, *Br. J. Obstet. Gynaec.*, 84, 165-74

Campbell, D. M., MacGillivray, I., Carr-Hill, R. and Samphier, M. (1983b). Fetal sex and pre-eclampsia in privigravidae, *Br. J. Obstet. Gynaec.*, 90, 26-27

Campbell, S. (1976). The antenatal assessment of fetal growth and development: the contribution of ultrasonic measurement. In: *The Biology of Human Fetal Growth* (ed. D. F. Roberts and A. M. Thomson), Taylor and Francis, London

Campbell, S. and Thoms, A. (1977). Ultrasound measurement of the head to abdomen circumference ratio in the assessment of growth retardation, *Br. J. Obstet. Gynaec.*, 84, 165-74

Carr-Hill, R. A. and Pritchard, C. W. (1983). Reviewing birthweight standards, *Br. J. Obstet. Gynaec.*, 90, 718

Carr-Hill, R. A. and Samphier, M. (1983). Birthweight and reproductive careers, *J. Biosoc. Sci.*, 15 (4), 453-64

Chamberlain, R. (1975). Birthweight and length of gestation. In: *British Births 1970* (ed. R. Chamberlain, G. Chamberlain, B. Howlett and A. Claireaux), Heinemann, London, pp. 45-88

Cheng, M. C. E., Chew, P. C. T. and Ratnam, S. S. (1972). Birthweight distribution of Singapore Chinese, Malay and Indian infants from 32 to 42 weeks gestation, *J. Obstet. Gynaec. Br. Commonw.*, 79, 149-53

Dawson, I., Golder, R. I. and Jonas, E. G. (1982). Birthweight by gestational age and its effect on perinatal mortality in white and Punjabi births: experience at a district hospital in West London 1967-1975, *Br. J. Obstet. Gynaec.*, 89, 896-99

DHSS (1980). Inequalities in health, *Black Report*, HMSO, London

Dobbing, J. and Sands, J. (1978). Head circumference, biparatal diameter and brain growth in fetal and postnatal life, *Early Hum. Dev.*, 2, 81-87

Donald, H. P. (1938-39). Sources of variation in human birth weights, *Proc. R. Soc., Edinburgh*, 59, 91-108

Dougherty, C. R. S. and Jones, A. D. (1982). The determinants of birth weight, *Am. J. Obstet. Gynec.*, 144, 190-200

Dowding, V. M. (1981). New assessment of the effects of birth order and socio-economic status on birth weight, *Br. med. J.*, 282, 683-86

Duffus, G. M. and MacGillivray, I. (1968). The incidence of pre-eclamptic toxaemia in smokers and non-smokers, *Lancet*, 1, 994-95

Duncan, O. D. (1975). *Introduction to Structural Equation Models*, Academic Press, New York

Dunlop, J. C. H. (1966). Chronic hypertension and perinatal mortality, *Proc. R. Soc. Med.*, 59, 838-41

Forbes, J.F. and Smalls, M.J. (1983). A comparative analysis of birthweight for gestational age standards, *Br. J. Obs. Gynaec.*, **99**, 297-303

Fraccaro, M. (1955). A contribution to the study of birthweight based on an Italian sample, *Am. Hum. Genet.*, **20**, 282-98

Fraccaro, M. (1958). Data for quantitative genetics in man. Birthweight in official statistics, *Human Biol.*, **30**, 142-49

Goldstein, M. S. (1947). Infants of Mexican descent: I. Physical status of neonates, *Child Develop.*, **18**, 3

Grimes, D. A. and Gross, G. K. (1981). Pregnancy outcomes in reproductive careers, *J. biosoc. Sci.*, **15**, 453-464

Gruenwald, P. (1966). Growth and maturation of the fetus and its relationship to perinatal mortality. In: *Perinatal Problems* (ed. N. R. Butler and E. D. Alberman), Livingstone, Edinburgh, pp. 141-62

Grundy, M. F. B., Hood, J. and Newman, G. B. (1978). Birthweight standards in a community of mixed racial origin, *Br. J. Obstet. Gynaec.*, **85**, 481-86

Hall, M., Campbell, D. M., Fraser, C., Carr-Hill, R. and Samphier, M. (1984). Extent and significance of uncertain gestations, *Br. J. Obstet. Gynaec.* (in press)

Hanushek, E. A. and Jackson, J. E. (1977). *Statistical Methods for Social Scientists*, Academic Press, New York

Hardy, J. B. (1969). Adverse fetal outcome following maternal rubella after the first trimester of pregnancy, *J. Am. med. Assoc.*, **207**, 2414-20

Haworth, J. C., Ellestad-Sayed, J. J., Kings, J. and Dilling, L. A. (1980). Relation of maternal cigarette smoking, obesity and energy consumption to infant size, *Am. J. Obstet. Gynec.*, **138**, 1185-89

Hellier, J. L. and Goldstein, H. (1979). The use of birthweight and gestation to assess perinatal mortality risk, *J. Epid. Comm. Hlth*, **33**, 183-85

Hendricks, C. H. (1964). Patterns of fetal and placental growth: the second half of normal pregnancy, *Obstet. Gynec.*, **24**, 357-65

Hendricks, C. H. (1967). Delivery patterns and reproductive efficiency among groups of differing socio-economic status and ethnic origins, *Am. J. Obstet. Gynec.*, **97**, 608-24

Hytten, F. E. and Leitch, I. (1971). *The Physiology of Human Pregnancy*, 2nd edn, Blackwells, Oxford

Illsley, R. (1955). Social class and selection, *Br. med. J.*, **II**, 15-20

Illsley, R. and Mitchell, R. G. (1984). *Low Birthweight: A Medical and Psychological Study*, John Wiley, Chichester

Jeliffe, E. F. P. (1968). Live birthweight and malarial infection of the placenta, *Bull. Wld Hlth Org.*, **38**, 69-78

Joreskog, K. G. and Sorbom, D. (1979). *Advances in Factor Analysis and Structural Analysis*, Abt. Books, Cambridge, Mass.

Joubert, D. M. and Hammond, J. (1954). Maternal effect on birthweight in South Devon and Dexter cattle crosses, *Nature Lond.*, **174**, 647-48

Karn, M. N. and Penrose, L. S. (1951). Birthweight and gestation time in relation to maternal age, parity and infant survival, *Ann. Eugen. (Lond.)*, 147-64

Kassius, R. V., Randall, A., Tompkins, W. T. and Wiehl, D. G. (1958). Maternal and newborn nutritional studies at Philadelphia lying-in hospital. Newborn studies. VI. Infant size at birth and parity, length of gestation, maternal age, height and weight status, *Milbank Memorial Fund Quarterly*, **36**, 335-62

Kettle, E. S. (1960). Weight and height curves for Australian Aboriginal infants and children, *Med. J. Aust.*, **1**, 972-77

Kloosterman, G. J. (1970). On intrauterine growth: the significance of perinatal care, *Int. J. Gynec. Obstet.*, **8**, 895-912

Leitch, I., Hytten, F. E. and Billewicz, W. Z. (1959). The maternal and neo-natal weights of some mammalia, *Proc. Zool. Soc. Lond.*, **133**, 11–28

Lette, R. and Fox, J. (1977). Registrar General's social classes: origins and uses, *Population Trends*, 7, HMSO

Levy, R. J., Rosenthal, A., Fyler, D. C. and Naclas, A. S. (1978). Birthweight of infants with congenital heart disease, *Am. J. Dis. Child.*, **132**, 249–54

Long, P. A., Abell, D. A. and Beischer, N. A. (1980). Fetal growth retardation and pre-eclampsia, *Br. J. Obstet. Gynaec.*, **65**, 536–39

Love, E. J. and Kinch, R. A. H. (1965). Factors affecting birthweight in normal pregnancy, *Am. J. Obstet. Gynec.*, **91**, 342–49

Lowe, C. R. (1961). Toxaemia and pre-pregnancy weight, *J. Obstet. Gynaec. Br. Commw.*, **68**, 622–27

Lubchenco, L. O., Hansman, C., Dressler, M. and Boyd, E. (1963). Intrauterine growth as estimated from live born birthweight data at 24 to 42 weeks gestation, *Pediatrics*, **32**, 793–800

Luke, B. and Petrie, R. H. (1980). Intrauterine growth: the correlation of infant birth weight and maternal post partem weight, *Am. J. Clin. Nutr.*, **33**, 2311–17

Lund, C. J. and Weese, W. H. (1953). Glucose tolerance and excessively large babies in non-diabetic mothers, *Am. J. Obstet. Gynec.*, **65**, 815–32

McCullough, R. E., Reeves, J. T. and Liljegren, R. L. (1977). Fetal growth retardation and increased infant mortality at high altitudes, *Arch. Environ. Hlth*, **32**, 26

McDonald, A. D. (1962). Early prenatal factors and prematurity, *J. Obstet. Gynaec. Br. Commw.*, **69**, 502–5

McEwan, H. P. and Murdoch, R. (1966). The oversized baby, a study of 169 cases, *J. Obstet. Gynaec. Br. Commw.*, **73**, 734–41

MacGillivray, I. (1967). The significance of blood pressure and body water changes in pregnancy, *Scot. med. J.*, **12**, 237–45

McKeown, T. and Record, R. G. (1954). Influence of pre-natal environment on the correlation between birthweight and parental height, *Am. J. Hum. Genet.*, **6**, 457–63

Meredith, H. V. (1970). Body weight at birth of viable human infants: a world-wide comparative treatise, *Human Biol.*, **42**, 217–64

Miller, H.C. and Hassanein, K. (1976). Fetal growth retardation in relation to maternal smoking and weight gain in pregnancy, *Am. J. Obstet. Gynec.*, **125**, 55–60

Miller, H. C., Hassanein, K. and Hensleigh, P. A. (1977). Effects of behavioural and medical variables on fetal growth retardation, *Am. J. Obstet. Gynec.*, **127**, 643–48

Miller, H. C., Hassanein, K. and Hensleigh, P. A. (1978). Maternal factors in the indices of low birthweight infants among black and white mothers, *Pediat. Res.*, **12**, 1016–19

Mills, J. and Seng, Y. P. (1954). The effect of age and parity of the mother on birthweight of the offspring, *Ann. Hum. Genet.*, **18**, 58–67

Milner, R. D. G. and Richards, B. (1974). An analysis of birthweight by gesta-tional age of infants born in England and Wales 1967–71, *J. Obstet. Gynaec. Br. Commw.*, **81**, 956–67

Moore, M. P. and Redman, C. W. G. (1983). Case-control study of severe pre-eclampsia of early onset, *Br. med. J.*, **287**, 6392, 580–83

Morton, N. E. (1955). The inheritance of human birthweight, *Ann. Hum. Genet.*, **20**, 125–34

Morton, N. E., Chung, C. S. and Mi, M. P. (1967). *Genetics of inter-racial crosses*

in Hawaii, Monographs in *Human Genetics*, Vol. 3, Karzer, New York
Mosely, D. and Knox, G. (1960). The birth weights of Yoruba babies, *J. Obstet. Gynaec. Br. Commw.*, **67**, 975–80
Naeye, R. L., Diener, M. M., Harcke, H. T. and Blanc, W. A. (1971). Relation of poverty and race to birthweight and organ cell structure in the newborn, *Pediat. Res.*, **5**, 17–22
Naeye, R. L. and Dixon, J. B. (1978). Distortions in fetal growth standards, *Pediat. Res.*, **12**, 987–91
Neligan, G. (1965). A community study of the relationships between birth weight and gestational age. In: *Clinics in Developmental Medicine, no. 19* (ed. M. Dawkins and W. G. MacGregor), Spastics Society and Heinemann, London, pp. 28–32
Nie, N. M. (1978). *Statistical Package for the Social Services*, McGraw-Hill, New York
Nie, N. M. (1980). *SPSS Update*, McGraw-Hill, New York
North, A. F., Mazundar, S. and Lozrillo, V. M. (1977). Birthweight, gestational age and perinatal deaths in 5,471 infants of diabetic mothers, *J. Pediat.*, **90**, 444–47
OECD (Organisation for Economic Co-operation and Development) (1976). Data sources for social indicators of victimisation suffered by individuals, *OECD Social Indicator Development Programme Special Study No. 3*, Paris
Osler, M. and Pedersen, J. (1960). The body composition of newborn infants of diabetic mothers, *Pediatrics*, **26**, 985–92
O'Sullivan, J. B., Gellis, S. S., Dandrow, R. V. and Tennay, B. D. (1966). The potential diabetic and her treatment in pregnancy, *Obstet. Gynec.*, **27**, 683–89
O'Sullivan, J. B., Charles, D., Mahan, C. M. and Dandrow, R. V. (1973). Gestational diabetics and perinatal mortality rate, *Am. J. Obstet. Gynec.*, **116**, 901–4
Ouellette, E.M., Rosett, H.L., Rossman, N.P. and Weiner, L. (1977). Adverse effects on offspring of maternal alcohol abuse during pregnancy, *New Engl. J. Med.*, **297**, 528–30
Page, E. W. and Christianson, R. (1976). Influence of blood pressure changes with and without proteinuria upon the outcome of pregnancy, *Am. J. Obstet. Gynec.*, **126**, 821–33
Papoz, L., Eschweze, E., Pequignot, G., Barratt, J. and Schwartz, D. (1982). Maternal smoking and birth weight in relation to dietary habits, *Am. J. Obstet. Gynec.*, **142**, 870–76
Pedersen, J. (1954). Weight and length at birth of infants of diabetic mothers, *Acta Endocr.*, **16**, 330–42
Pirani, B. B. K. (1978). Smoking during pregnancy, *Obstet. Gynec. Surv.*, **33**, 1–13
Pritchard, C.W. and Thompson, B. (1982). Starting a family in Scotland, *J. Biosoc. Sci.*, **14**, 2
Pritchard, C. W., Sutherland, H. and Carr-Hill, R. (1983). Birthweight and paternal height, *Br. J. Obstet. Gynaec.*, **90**, 156–61
Register General (1981). *Classification of Occupations*, HMSO, London
Roberts, D.F. (1976). Environment and the fetus. In: *The Biology of Human Fetal Growth* (ed. D.F. Roberts and A.M. Thomson), Taylor and Francis, London, p. 271
Robson, E. B. (1955). Birthweight in cousins, *Ann. Human Genet.*, **19**, 262–67
Rush, D. Davies, H. and Susser, M. (1972). Antecedents of low birthweight in Harlem, New York City, *Int. J. Epidemiol.*, **1**, 375–87

Rush, D., Davies, H. and Susser, M. (1980). A randomised controlled trial of prenatal nutritional supplementation in New York City, *Paediatrics*, **65**, 683–97

Samphier, M. and Thompson, B. (1982). The Aberdeen maternity and neonatal data bank. In: *Prospective Longitudinal Research* (ed. S. A. Medrick and A. E. Baert), OUP, London

Scott, K. E. and Usher, R. (1966). Fetal malnutrition: its incidence, causes and effects, *Am. J. Obstet. Gynec.*, **94**, 951–63

Selvin, S. and Janerich, D. T. (1971). Four factors influencing birthweight, *Br. J. prev. soc. Med.*, **25**, 12–16

Sibert, J. R., Jadav, M. and Indaraj, S. G. (1978). Maternal and fetal nutrition in South India, *Br. med. J.*, **1**, 1517–18

Smith, C. A. (1947). Effects of maternal under-nutrition upon the newborn infant in Holland, 1944–45, *J. Pediat.*, **30**, 229–43

Sobrevilla, L. A., Romero, I., Kruger, F. and Whittembury, J. (1968). Low oestrogen excretion during pregnancy at high altitude, *Am. J. Obstet. Gynec.*, **102**, 828–33

Stein, Z. and Susser, M. (1975). The Dutch famine 1944–45 and the reproductive process. *Pediat. Res.*, **9**, 70

Stevenson, R. E. (1977). Prenatal infections. In: *The Fetus and Newly Born Infant: Influences of the Prenatal Environment*, C. V. Mosby Co., St Louis, pp. 195–333

Stewart, A. and Hewitt, D. (1960). Toxaemia of pregnancy and obesity, *J. Obstet. Gynaec. Br. Emp.*, **67**, 812–18

Sutherland, H. W., Stowers, J. M. and Mckenzie, C. (1970). Simplifying the clinical problem of glycosuria in pregnancy, *Lancet*, **1**, 1069–71

Tennes, K. and Blackard, C. (1980). Maternal alcohol consumption, birth weight and minor physical anomalies, *Am. J. Obstet. Gynec.*, **138**, 774–80

Thomson, A. M. (1957). Technique and perspective in clinical and dietary studies of human pregnancy, *Br. J. Nutr.*, **13**, 509–25

Thomson, A. M. (1971). Physiological determinants of birthweight, *Proc. 2nd European Congress of Perinatal Medicine*, Karger, Basel, pp. 174–80

Thomson, A. M. (1983). Fetal size at birth. In: *Obstetrical Epidemiology* (ed. S.L. Barron and A.M. Thomson), Academic Press, London

Thomson, A. M. and Billewicz, W. Z. (1976). The concept of the light for dates infant. In: *The Biology of Human Fetal Growth* (ed. D. F. Roberts and A. M. Thomson), Taylor and Francis, London

Thomson, A. M., Hytten, F. E. and Billewicz, W. Z. (1967). The epidemiology of oedema during pregnancy, *J. Obstet. Gynaec. Br. Commw.*, **74**, 1–10

Thomson, A.M., Billewicz, W.Z. and Hytten, F.E. (1968). The assessment of fetal growth, *J. Obstet. Gynaec. Br. Commw.*, **75**, 903–16

Tompkins, W. T., Wiehl, D. G. and Mitchell, R. M. (1955). The underweight patient as an increased obstetric hazard, *Am. J. Obstet. Gynec.*, **69**, 114–23

Underwood, P., Hester, L. L., Lafette, T. and Gregg, K. V. (1965). The relationship of smoking to the outcome of pregnancy, *Am. J. Obstet. Gynec.*, **91**, 270–76

United States Public Health Service (1979). *Smoking and Health: A Report of the Surgeon General*, Department of Health and Welfare, Washington, D.C.

Usher, R. and Maclean, F. (1969). Intrauterine growth of live born Caucasian infants at sea-level: standards obtained from measurements in 7 dimensions of infants born between 25 and 44 weeks of gestation, *J. Pediat.*, **74**, 901–10

Usher, R. H. and Maclean, F. H. (1974). Normal fetal growth and the significance of fetal growth retardation. In: *Scientific Foundations of Paediatrics* (ed.

J. A. Davies and J. Dobbing), Heinemann, London, pp. 69–80

Vedra, B. and Pavlikova, E. (1969). Onset of abnormal weight gain in pre-eclamptic pregnancy, *J. Obst. Gynaec. Br. Commw.*, **76**, 873

Walton, A. and Hammond, J. (1938). The maternal effects on growth and conformation in Shire horse–Shetland pony crosses, *Proc. R. Soc.*, **125B**, 311–35

Wilcox, A. J. (1981). Birthweight gestation and the fetal growth curve, *Am. J. Obstet. Gynec.*, **139** (8), 863–67

Workshop on Nutrition of the Child (1981). Maternal Nutritional Status and Fetal Outcome, Report of Proceedings, *Am. J. Clin. Nutr.*, **34**

Yamazaki, J. W., Wright, S. W. and Wright, P. M. (1954). Outcome of pregnancy in women exposed to the atomic bomb in Nagasaki, *Am. J. Dis. Child*, 87, 448–63

Yerushalmy, J. (1971). The relationship of parents' cigarette smoking to outcome of pregnancy – implications as to the problems of inferring causation from observed associations, *Am. J. Epidemiol.*, **93**, 443–56

Yerushalmy, J. (1972). Infants of low birthweight born before their mothers started to smoke cigarettes, *Am. J. Obstet. Gynec.*, **112**, 277–84

Yerushalmy, J. (1974). Cigarette smoking, infant birthweight and perinatal mortality rates, *Am. J. Obstet. Gynec.*, **118**, 884–86

Name Index*

*See also the References on pages 181–187.

Subject Index